Your Phone Can Save Your Life

How <u>You</u> Can Benefit From The Biggest Revolution In The History Of Medicine

by
David Kerrigan

Disclaimer

All content within this book or referenced is provided for general information only, and should not be treated as a substitute for the medical advice of your own doctor or any other health care professional. The author or publisher is not responsible or liable for any diagnosis made by a reader based on the content of this book. The author/publisher is not liable for the contents of any external internet sites listed, nor does it endorse any commercial product or service mentioned on any of the sites. **Always consult a healthcare professional if you're in any way concerned about your health and do not make any changes to your lifestyle without first consulting a healthcare professional.**

Acknowledgements

This book is dedicated to my parents and brother.
My thanks to all my friends who encouraged me to complete this book especially Aideen, Caroline, Lorraine, Susan, Sylvia, Adam, Fergal, Ken, Rob and Simon.

For More Information

Visit the website: http://www.yourphonecansaveyourlife.com

Contents

Chapters

Appendices

Chapter 1: Introduction

My mobile phone knows more about my health than my doctor does. And for the first time in my life, I know more about my own well-being than just feeling "well", "ok" or "sick". I know that my blood pressure is normal, my temperature is normal, my heart rate is normal, my blood oxygen level is normal and my ECG shows no abnormalities, yet I haven't been to a doctor in years. I also know I get the recommended amount of exercise every day, eat the appropriate amount of calories and don't usually get quite enough sleep - all with scientific detail that has never before been available outside of a clinical setting.

All this isn't because I live in some parallel future universe, am insanely wealthy or have employed a team of doctors, personal trainers and nutritionists. It's entirely possible to collect all of this information with easy to use off-the-shelf products that cost just a few hundred pounds. All this is possible because I've embraced just some of the vast array of features, apps and accessories that are now available in conjunction with my phone to focus on improving my well-being, even to the point of extending my life expectancy.

Having access to information that could extend your life is really quite profound, and has not yet received the kind of widespread attention I believe it deserves, and rather than wait around for it to take its inevitable course over the coming years of gradually coming to prominence, I am going to spend the rest of this book trying to provide a shortcut guide to make the whole topic more accessible.

"We've gone through an extraordinary revolution over the last five years, but sometimes when you're in the middle of fundamental change it is hard to spot."

- Rory Cellan-Jones, Technology Correspondent, BBC.

1

A Phone Is Not Just A Phone

Quietly unnoticed and masquerading under the simple guise of a phone, the key to the biggest revolution in healthcare since antibiotics is now in the pockets and handbags of over half the population in most developed countries. The impact that these and related technologies is about to have on our health is unprecedented. This book will guide you through what's happening and show you how you can benefit, if you choose to.

As recently as just 3 or 4 years ago, the biggest contribution your phone could make to your well-being was calling for help in an emergency. While it can still do that, it can now play an active role in reducing the likelihood you'll have to call them. It's time to stop thinking of it as a phone and start to look at it as a personal computer: the first true personal computer. The personal computers that came to prominence in the 1980s and 1990s were personal only in that they were available for individual use. So the smartphone is really the first true personal computer - a computer that is personal not only in the sense of being a computer that just one individual uses and you carry it with you, but also in that it provides information about your person. In 1982, Time Magazine declared the Personal Computer as "Machine of the Year". It was without doubt the beginning of an era where ordinary individuals had unprecedented access to computing power that could be harnessed to their own ends instead of corporate computational tasks. But the true personal computer is now in the shape of the smartphone. It knows plenty about us (much more than we may realize), and tackles organization, communication, navigation, entertainment, medical and other duties. Mobiles are the true personal computers with stunning power, ease of use and even affordability in a package that fits in your pocket.

Of course no revolution the scale of which we're investigating here comes without its challenges. This book is not a technologically-apologetic view that sees a panacea or automated elixir. Some of the problems facing the future of healthcare are very real and will take enormous effort to overcome. Others are less daunting and result primarily from entrenched views or ignorance rather than fundamental or insurmountable issues. But it's now time for more people to be aware of the opportunities emerging and to have an informed rational debate about how best to seize the positives and minimize or eliminate the negatives. The ground-breaking health dividend that is within our grasp should be made available to the widest possible audience.

Finding Your Solutions

Although technology has already started reshaping so many of our daily interactions, it's not surprising that an area as traditional and complex as healthcare has lagged behind. But as we'll see, technology is now readily available to democratize access to healthcare information and solutions are appearing that address the very personal nature of health. There will be pressure from consumers too - people used to digital interactions in every other industry that has been swept by technology (air travel, banking, education and shopping) will be puzzled when health professionals don't speak their language. So-called "Digital Natives" will not tolerate analog customer service for something as crucial as their health.

There is no one-size fits all solution to the provision of healthcare and in many cases health-related beliefs and lifestyle choices may be firmly rooted in social, religious or political contexts - the responses to new approaches will vary across age, socio-economic groups and be influenced by cultural or ideological beliefs. You may already have some fairly entrenched views about many of the topics in the coming pages but I ask that you put aside your preconceptions for just a few hours.

Whatever your preferences for medical care, be they traditional, holistic, alternative or other, I am not either advocating or rejecting such approaches. In fact, this book is mainly about prevention, detection and monitoring, not about cure: choosing treatments remains firmly something for you and your chosen healthcare professional, albeit it likely increasingly influenced by technology.

Yet this is not about blindly believing that technology will solve all ills. Common sense must prevail and people need to see the combined benefits of technology alongside the importance of human experience. Over-reliance on technology at the expense of human intuition and intelligence will lead to ill-considered outcomes in many cases. I in no way want to medicalize every day issues, nor resort to science-y sounding claims to give extra credence to what I say, but I do want to aim to create a firmly evidentiary basis for assessing the benefits or otherwise of the various technologies, hence any references to the scientific basis for the technologies discussed.

Throughout this book, the cost of bad health is mentioned several times. Whether you measure this cost in lost lives, ill-health or cold hard cash, it's worth stopping to consider the scale of what we're talking about. Like it or not, 3 out of 4 people do not currently adhere to recommended healthy lifestyle choices. I do not want to be alarmist or scare people unnecessarily but some of the options presented are pretty stark. There are no guarantees, and of course there are numerous other factors, but those who make clearly negligent choices regarding their lifestyle may soon face stringent financial consequences as well as increased risks of negative outcomes. And by negative outcomes I mean serious illness or death. Undoubtedly some people will choose to live life in a way that suits them, whatever the potential influence on outcomes. And so it should be in a world of freedom, but they may not be able to rely on other people to continue to pay for it indefinitely, as correlations and causation evidence are combined with monitoring and compliance technologies to identify where and when people are not taking reasonable precautions.

It is very important to look at the actual problems that I'm suggesting technology can help to address - this is very much not about technology just for the sake of it. I've tried to look at the impacts in question and not get drawn into monitoring only the surrogate outcomes - Dr Ben Goldacre has written extensively on this concept as a classic example of how Bad Science can take hold. For example, measuring reductions in blood pressure is not an end in itself - the desired outcome is a measurable drop in death from heart attacks attributed to high blood pressure. Sure, blood pressure may be a contributory factor but it's important to remember the real reason you may undertake a change in your lifestyle - not to change just an indicator but to affect a very real preferential outcome of living longer!

The Times They Are A-Changing

I've found myself amazed by technology more in the last 5 or 6 years than in the previous 15. If you haven't been looking (and most people haven't), the technologies described in this book as now being routinely and affordably available on the high street may seem to have come from nowhere. Yet much of the technology has been available in one form or another for a few years. There hasn't been one big advance in technology but a succession/combination of several things - the proliferation of phones that has placed computing power previously beyond imagination in every pocket, the adoption of apps which give one-touch access to dedicated systems, Bluetooth Low Energy which allows short range data synchronization without harming battery life, and technologies such as Application Programming Interfaces (API) that enable easy integration of disparate systems. The range of items you can measure now in your own home would have been beyond the imagination of a doctor only a few years ago. In fact, a few hundred dollars' worth of "appcessories" (a piece of hardware that requires an app to work) would rival the diagnostic testing capabilities of a small doctor's surgery. This trend will likely only accelerate.

Much of the technology described in the book - hardware or software apps - will change before this volume is even published. But the specific models available today are not the focus of the book. I have taken examples of current technology to illustrate what's currently on the market but the key point is the seismic shift in the availability and pace of change of technology that empowers people to become more active than ever before in managing their own health and well-being more.

Objective

The aim of this book is twofold - 1. to help people understand the range of easy to use, affordable technologies that now exist to help support anyone who wants to lead a healthier lifestyle. And 2, to discuss some of the significant changes and challenges posed by the emergence of these technologies. It is not aimed specifically at technical or medical audiences and will be easily understood by anyone who doesn't have a special interest in technology or health matters but has a desire to improve their well-being. It tries to guide the reader through the plethora of devices now emerging that purport to offer significant new opportunities to take an active role in understanding or managing their health and well-being. It also addresses the changes that such new tools may catalyze in the medical arena and adjacent sectors. But make no mistake: these trends are not here to replace doctors but to enable patients who want to, to be better informed and to have a more collaborative approach to their health outcomes.

I hope it provides a practical guide to understand the rapidly changing technology that may help you make an informed choice about what might work for you and enable you to have a conversation with your physician to determine if there is a regime you should consider implementing. It may help to Identify some life-improving opportunities that you might otherwise miss. Of course you may decide it's not for you, and that's fine, but better you know and choose not to than not know about the advances that might take away some of the barriers that previously impeded your adoption of health-supporting practices.

It's perhaps helpful at this point to be explicit about what this book is and isn't about. For example, this book is not a weight-loss guide. Sure, you may lose weight if you employ the food monitoring techniques described and/or undertake the levels of activities that the various methods available might suggest. But to be clear, technology alone will not make you lose weight. All it can do is help you understand, motivate you and perhaps get some support from friends if that's what appeals to you.

This is also not buyer's guide for specific devices - I reference examples here by necessity to illustrate the range and versatility of the offerings available today but the pace of change dictates that any attempt at a buyer's guide in printed format will be obsolete long before it hits the shelves, even if they are virtual shelves. And that's a good thing. While it may prove a little intimidating to someone trying to choose how to invest in their health, it also shows that pace of change and improvement in these devices is relentless. To be clear, no company was given the opportunity to comment on or influence the conclusions regarding specific devices - I have included a fairly representative sample of popular devices, but cannot include every product. The omission of a specific device in no way implies it is sub-standard, just as the inclusion of a device does not imply a recommendation. I hope that the broad overview of what is available will arm the interested consumer with sufficient knowledge to make an informed decision on the types of technology that may be of benefit to them in taking a proactive interest in their health.

You may conclude that the time is not right for you to purchase a health device and that's okay. I would readily admit that some of the gadgets I've tried in the last year while researching this book were absolutely not ready for mass market use as they suffered from teething problems. But that's an important part of the development cycle and many of these products can only develop when they are tested by large numbers of consumers in the real world, who can contribute information and insights to guide the evolution of these gadgets.

Yet a surprising number of solutions are what I would consider "consumer ready". They reliably do what they claim, provide actionable data and are easy to use. Yet I have no doubt that the devices I am looking at today will be radically different in as little as two years' time. They will be smaller, lighter, cheaper and have better battery life while including more features. But such is the way of technology and the best advice I can offer is that you choose the product that best suits your health needs at the time rather than waiting for the next version that will undoubtedly be better.

Along with devices, there's a similarly bewildering array of apps and accessories that purport to revolutionize your life. I want to demystify these and examine the role each could play in your life. There is no one size fits all solution (yet) and despite the over exuberant claims of the various suppliers, I haven't found any that work without a liberal dose of motivation and application.

It Doesn't Have To End Here

Many of the topics I cover relatively briefly here would merit a book in their own right. And where you're interested in a more in-depth view on a particular topic, I have highlighted in Appendix B some books or sources that I have found to be insightful. If the discussions in this book pique your interest in the bigger picture beyond your own well-being it might even inform a few discussions with your public representatives to pressure them into health service reform. Remember that it's very unlikely that at some point in your life you won't come into contact with your national health service so it's a good idea to do what you can to shape it before you need it, rather than wait until your hour of need to realize that it's not what you were expecting.

I firmly believe that it would be a shame for any person who could benefit in any way from exposure to these technologies to miss out through lack of awareness or information. And so I hope that by the end of this book you may have enough information to move forward with a degree of confidence, safe in the knowledge that you are not starting from scratch and have answers to your most basic questions. Remember, this is neither a technology book nor a medical book; it's a people book. It's about ensuring that people have access to information about the technologies available today that might improve their well-being, if they choose to use them.

I will follow a similar layout for each section - what is the problem, what are the underlying technologies and what are the kinds of solutions available today. I hope that this enables you to assess the applicability of the topic and its potential suitability, if any, in your own life. I have tried not to get too technical either in medical or electronic terms but I trust that this is an important enough topic that you may take the time to understand in a little more detail the topics being discussed. I am aiming to find the middle ground between dumbing down and over medicalization or sensationalization.

My hope is that a proportion of people reading this book will decide to give technology a try and find it helps them to better health. I am what is termed a technology optimist. I believe that technology can make the world a better place if used correctly. And if it's widely enough available, affordable and people are aware of it. I'm not a technology apologist who believes that technology is the answer to all human ills - all I want is for people to be informed about the changes that have taken place in the last few years and to judge for themselves if they want to harness these advances for their personal benefit. I will not label those who don't as luddites, but want to raise the point that health services or health insurers around the world may soon penalize those who don't take a more active interest in their own well-being.

If just a few people were to find a way to better manage a chronic condition or even if this helped one person discover an issue earlier than they would otherwise, to me that's a good result.

How Important Is Your Health To You?

We humans are not always rational creatures. Given how strong our survival instinct is when faced with a clear and present danger, we respond very differently when the danger is less clear or less imminent. When asked if health is important to them, the vast majority of people say yes. But when asked how much time or effort they put into staying healthy or avoiding behaviors that are known to be harmful, the positive answers fall sharply.

A lot of people are fascinated by medical drama. For years, the most popular shows in the US have included ER, House MD and Grey's Anatomy, while UK audiences add Casualty and Holby City to the mix. Yet while these fictional shows command our attention, we are strangely indifferent to our own well-being unless it is acutely bothering us. Most people invest very little time in their health. Until it goes wrong. We actually know remarkably little about ourselves beyond a feeling of 'not quite right' and commonly a tendency to overestimate our malady. We also act irrationally or try to persuade ourselves nothing's wrong for fear that it is, or that investigation might prove painful or expensive. For a variety of reasons people aren't very proactive about their health. They bring their car for a service once a year, expect it to require some care/attention to pass its MOT but when it comes to their own well-being, most visit a doctor only when something is clearly wrong. This may be caused by a lack of time, a lack of compulsion (this may change as insurance companies and eventually national healthcare requires it), a lack of money, a lack of accessibility or a fear of doctors. Technology is ideally placed to address many if not all of these barriers.

We will talk in the following chapters about illnesses and diseases with varying degrees of seriousness - from the casual or cosmetic through the management of serious chronic medical conditions to the life changing or worse. Let's be clear upfront though - impressive as the technologies emerging to combat these may be; none is a substitute for professional medical advice. All of the technologies presented here are intended to inform, motivate and assist both people and healthcare professionals, or to streamline processes and tasks - not replace common sense, professional wisdom and experience. The rest of this book will focus on apps and accessories with a strong mobile element. There are of course numerous web sites, services and forums to learn more about illness that do not have any dedicated mobile element and while these are in many cases very useful, often run by official bodies such as the NHS, it is the personal and persistent nature of the mobile phone and its associated services that are defining a new era in personal health management. Let's start with a brief look at the technologies that are enabling this era and how they've come to create so much opportunity so quickly.

Chapter 2:
Standing Still Is Not An Option

Any sufficiently advanced technology is indistinguishable from magic

- Arthur C Clarke

In the 1990 book The Machine that Changed the World, the car and Japanese lean production was singled out as the most significant industrial advance of the 20th century. Although we're barely 15 years into the 21st century, it seems very likely that the smartphone is the early runaway contender for the next title. In fact, if self-driving cars come to fruition (and there are already Google cars in daily autonomous action on the roads of California), the machine that changed the world last century will be controlled by the machine that changed the world this century.

Before we delve into the application of technologies for health and well-being purposes, I just want to spend a few minutes to highlight the recent advances that make the rest of this book even possible. What has happened in the last decade or so that seemingly almost by accident has brought us to his point? As is so often the case, the advances that we now can apply to our health did not begin life intended to make us better. But the ingenious application of technologies in fields beyond their original design, coupled with decreasing size and cost and increasing power, open up spectacular new possibilities.

In technology circles, the concept of Moore's Law refers to the prediction that computing power doubles approximately every 2 years. The progress this has delivered has been astonishing in the last few decades - computers today are about 1 trillion times faster than those of half a decade ago. The Apple Watch has twice the processing power of a 1980s Cray Supercomputer that took up a small room, yet it sits on your wrist and weighs a tad over 40 grams. Just 10 years ago, the smartphone didn't exist. 5 years ago, the iPad didn't exist. Now there are more mobile phones in the world than toothbrushes, and speaking of toothbrushes, the processor in my smart toothbrush is more powerful than a 1980s supercomputer!

It is very easy to forget that every time you leave the house, you are taking multiple sensors with you as well as having a device that only twenty years ago would have been the size of a room and cost about $10m. The decreasing size of transistor components means that during the iPhone 6 launch weekend in 2015, Apple sold 25 times more transistors than were in all of the personal computers on the entire planet just 20 years ago. The average user (thankfully) has no need to appreciate the fact that the chip inside their phone now contains around 2 billion transistors. We each individually now carry more computing power in our pocket than the entirety of NASA had at its disposal to send man to the moon.

After the years of rapid specification advances, we have now reached something of a smartphone plateau with smaller year on year changes in technical specifications. Manufacturers have made phones as thin as you can hold and put cameras in them that turn out results indistinguishable to most people from expensive SLR cameras. So rather than extolling the pure hardware advances of every upgrade, attention is turning to the role of these personal portable connected computers where they provide a central, coordinating locus of our digital lives. Sure, speeds will continue to advance, but the core capabilities are relatively stable for now. And this is a good thing - the emphasis now shifts to what we do with them rather than a focus on incremental technical specifications that deliver small end user benefits. We are at a point where most of them are fast enough as a basic platform that we can look at what they enable. The underlying speeds will continue to improve but the lowest common denominator is no longer very low.

With Great Power...

The important thing is how we choose to use all this processing power, sensor outputs and the applications enabled by the reductions in cost and size of technology. Coupled with advances and cost reductions in sensors, the power now available to us is transformative - if we choose to use it in the most efficient ways. Only seven or eight years ago, the notion that you could have a miniature computer in your pocket for a few hundred dollars that would also monitor your health would have been utterly far-fetched.

While we marvel at the advancement of smartphones as the most visible modern gadget, they don't exist in a vacuum - their potential usefulness is derived not only from their raw computing power, but their ability to communicate with other devices and services and access additional capabilities via software. This communication is via WiFi and mobile data networks providing fast Internet access from virtually everywhere, as well as Bluetooth providing short range connections to accessories. When you can't see it, it can be easy to take things for granted. The twin wireless communication technologies of WiFi and Bluetooth are crucial enablers to glue together the multitude of devices and services that make up the personal well-being ecosystem that's emerging. It's less than 15 years since I got the first Bluetooth headset you could buy (it cost around 15 times what Bluetooth headsets cost today) and there was only one phone that it worked with. Now Bluetooth is in virtually every phone and in millions of smart devices. My weighing scales connects to my phone via Bluetooth and uses WiFi to connect to the Internet, but more on that later. We take it for granted that we can send information from one device to another without having to connect them physically or even be in the same room as them. Without these invisible technologies, we would not be seeing the very visible progress of the last few years.

And although the first iPhone didn't even have an App Store, we are now all familiar with app stores that provide a simple distribution channel for innovative software. Anyone looking for software to help them with virtually any task can instantly search the millions of apps available, complete with user ratings for each of them to help you find not only one that claims to do what you want, but comes with recommendations to help you gauge its capabilities.

Despite the rapid pace at which affordable technologies are appearing on the market, it's worth acknowledging that producing this kind of technology is not easy. Creating good hardware that people can live with every day is difficult. It now involves a complex mix of design, fashion, battery life challenges, connectivity and robustness - anything attached to you is likely to get knocks, get wet and get exposed to hot and cold. Despite the monumental technological advances of the last couple of years that enable a company to put a device on our wrist for $15 that measures movement and sleep, communicates wirelessly with our phone, has a battery that lasts nearly two months per charge and is so waterproof you can swim with it, it's still hard to make functional and attractive wearable devices. Ones with screens and additional functions reduce the battery life from weeks or months to just hours or a day. More than one prominent activity tracker has been withdrawn from the market after reports of skin irritation. Yet I have no doubt that the pace of innovation will mean that in just a couple of years, these challenges will have been overcome - consumer electronics companies are good at overcoming these hard challenges and they will refine their products quickly to make the current ones look ridiculous, much as the mobile phone from 10 years ago look absurd beside today's.

On Demand Convenience

When you take a moment to consider how relatively new much of the technology we take for granted is, you start to realize just how rapidly technical capabilities are evolving, just as prices drop and sizes get smaller. We very quickly take convenience for granted. Reading a book recently about the founder of Amazon, the little fact that Kindle E-Readers didn't exist just six years ago jumped out as a good example that I hadn't realized. They cost

400 dollars when launched but now start at just $90. You see them in use in every age group every day. In fact, we now take for granted the fact we can instantly purchase and start reading virtually any book in the world from anywhere in the world. Just six years ago you couldn't. The great advances in convenience and consumption facilitated by technology have changed expectations about the speed at which we can access goods and services in most industries. Bill Gates' second book, Business at the Speed of Thought was published in 1999 and spoke of the Digital Nervous System that would transform business. In it, he advocated using information technology to release information to enable quantum leaps in efficiency, growth and profits. He compared business to a living organism and concluded his chapter on healthcare with the stark question "are you preparing for the day in the near future when patients insist on communicating over the web?". The millions of people now using online medical services suggest that day is upon us.

Finding the Way: Missteps to Democracy

Transformative technologies take time to find their place and usually end up somewhere between the most positive and most negative forecasts. Even the great Socrates was worried about the negative impact of writing and at various times through history many scholars opposed Printing, TV and numerous other developments. But all have eventually found their place in society, though not always as envisaged by their creators. With the physical and financial barriers to technology being removed, the availability and use of previously restricted specialist equipment is being democratized.

Just how far it can and should extend is a matter for debate and one of the central themes of this book. The perception of technology and its application changes over time and mistakes will undoubtedly be made before we reach the ultimate outcome. Just because a technology can be made available does not always mean that it should be, or that it will be used appropriately. My parents tell stories of how their local shoe shop once offered a service where they x-rayed children's feet to check the fit of a shoe. Now unthinkable, the concept of an x-ray machine being used without any medical supervision or radiation shielding was normal at the time. In that instance, the democratization of technology was definitely not a good thing!

The medical sector has benefitted from some huge technological advances in the last few decades, particularly in the area of imaging with devices like the MRI scanner. Sequencing of the first human genome took a decade and cost $3 billion but you can now do it for a $1,000 in slightly less than 48 hours. But while massive research projects and hospital equipment may have changed, the democratization and consumerization of technology that we've seen in other sectors has only just arrived. We will need to be careful not to confuse on-demand with urgent in an age of instant gratification.

Democratizing access is generally a good thing. It is historically accompanied by a period of turbulence as people re-adjust to the new power relationships before settling down. Equally, as medicine's "Gutenberg moment" unfolds, substantial educational and cultural structures need to be established for patients and clinicians alike. Printing presses might have made books more widely available, but people needed to learn how to read before the technology could truly be impactful. Similarly, technology might be democratizing healthcare, but people need to know how to work with those new dynamics.

The Future is Present

Clichés are phrases that are true but have lost their impact because we are so tired of hearing them. Take "The only constant is change" for example. But for anyone who thinks that things will stay as they are or that somehow the medical arena can resist the change that has swept other sectors, it's sobering to think that 429 of the original Fortune 500 companies from 1955 are no longer in business today. 429 of 500 of the world's largest companies gone, despite their impressive scale, resources and apparent power in just 60 years! With such change possible in a generation without us particularly noticing, what else is likely to shape our lives in the coming years? In a saying attributed to former President of the Institute for the Future and now known as Amara's Law, Roy Amara noted, "*We tend to overestimate the effect of a technology in the short run and underestimate the effect in the long run*". So many of the changes I point out as underway or possible may be dismissed by commentators as irrelevant if they don't take hold fast enough in this age of instant gratification. Yet it is likely that even larger changes than I am highlighting will actually take place within the space of just a few decades.

There are two reasons I'm not going to make too many predictions about the exact future evolution of technologies - primarily because I want to focus on what's already available, or will be available in the short term, that can start to help people now rather than waiting for the next iteration or breakthroughs that will inevitably come. And secondly, because predicting the future accurately when describing technology is really, really hard! Historic examples - like the President of IBM (in)famously predicting that global demand for computers might amount to a worldwide total of about five - serve as a warning to anyone getting into the future gazing game. And much more recently, a reminder that predicting the pace of change is not easy: Academics Levy & Murane from Harvard and MIT predicted in their 2004 book "The New Division of Labor" that driverless cars were not coming anytime soon. Yet barely 8 years later, you could be passed on a highway by a Google car driving without human intervention. In fairness to them, mobile phones of the day didn't yet routinely have touch screens or cameras - the pace of change can catch even the most techno-optimists off guard.

So I am not going to suggest specific timelines when things will happen. I will predict that less expensive phones will soon have health and wellness features, while high end phones will soon have more diagnostic capabilities than a well-equipped clinic has today. Soon is my way of saying I don't know exactly when in the next couple of years so I don't want to look too foolish. Wearables may one day in the not too distant future become implantables but I'm happy to leave that to the scientists to work on for now and concentrate on the solutions already available.

As I've said, future gazing/tech-prophesying is notoriously difficult and most usually wrong. But for me the measure of success is not picking the exact technology that will prevail, nor the precise timeframe in which things may change, but stimulating a debate about the pros and cons of technology enhanced life and thereby making people more aware. If this book serves only to help a few more people make an informed decision to embrace or eschew available technology, then I'll be satisfied. Access to technology and information about technology in a digestible format is crucial. It is virtually impossible for people to be aware of all of the emerging technologies that are available to help them improve their well-being. Despite the decreasing cost, it is likely that many people will be denied access on the basis of lack of knowledge or confusion.

I do believe that the current wave of technological development will be known as the Smart Age when future historians come to label us. The next significant age after the industrial age. And unlike that epoch, it's not one single technology that is dominant but parallel developments and new applications of these developments that define this era. Computer chips, networking technologies, wireless communications, apps, sensors and reducing prices all play a part.

Just as we can point to list a host of transformative health technologies from past generations such as antibiotics, x-rays and vaccinations, I hope that in the future, someone reviewing our current time and the near future will be able to reflect on it as having delivered even more examples of progress. There are numerous exciting and promising areas of advancement in medicine and treatments that are outside the scope of this book, as I seek only to highlight the impact of mobile-centric advances and opportunities. Exoskeletons, 3d printing of artificial organs and prosthetics as well as projects to give sight to the blind are the stuff of science fiction that also seem to be within our grasp in the near future.

Even if we haven't thought about it specifically, we all expect medical technology to improve and are impatient for it to do so when we or someone we care about needs medical assistance - how many people would have accepted it if Star Trek's Dr. McCoy still carried a stethoscope? We were impressed but not necessarily surprised when that vision of the future saw a handheld scanning device that diagnosed people in an instant. The good news is that we don't have to wait until the 23rd century for it to come true. The first rudimentary tricorder like device (if rudimentary is a fair word to apply to this remarkable device) is already available and I have no doubt that in less than 10 years' time, we will be looking at regular doctors with a device true to the Start Trek vision of the future. We'll talk about that device in the next chapter.

Measuring Technology

Keeping track of the adoption of personal technology is not going to be simple - it used to be quite easy to see statistically how well connected a country was - but increasingly it will be hard to know exactly how connected people are becoming. The traditional measure of mobile penetration (cellular connections per population) is clearly no longer going to be sufficient. While multiple device ownership and/or Machine to Machine (M2M - devices like smart meters or security cameras) have pushed most developed countries over the 100% mark, a more useful measure now must include the Bluetooth and WiFi connected devices that mask the actual number of devices connected by a single subscriber. A single subscriber may have an activity tracker, heart rate monitor and a connected scales all using their phone to access cloud storage and analysis services. Using old metrics, they would appear no more connected than a person with a single 2G phone. But the average household in the developed world has more phones than people, multiple televisions, several computers and tablets and probably a games console.

Among the technology that permeates our residences, there is often only one dedicated health-care related accessory - the thermometer. Maybe a bathroom scale. But that's about it. For most people, the medicine cabinet stacked with a few over the counter cold remedies, painkillers and maybe some prescription tablets is the sum total of our investment in our health. The modern medicine cabinet, as you'll see by the end of this book, will bear little resemblance to the collection of pill bottles of old. It will be replaced by smart technology, and the pill bottles will be delivered to us just in time, and apps will offer personalized advice in real time based on numerous sensors.

The Rise of Apps

The App may well become the single most prominent purveyor of well-being information and management. Over 100 billion apps have been downloaded from Apple's app store in just 7 years. According to Google, the fastest growing category of apps on Android in 2014 was Health & Fitness. Throughout this book, I highlight specific apps that serve to illustrate points I wanted to make. This is in no way a comprehensive guide to all the well-being apps that are available. There are simply too many for that! According to recent data, there are more than 100,000 Health apps currently available across multiple platforms on the global market. Approximately 70% of these apps target the consumer wellness and fitness segments; 30% target health professionals, easing access to patient data, patient consultation and monitoring, diagnostic imaging, pharmaceuticals information etc.

When combined with the information collecting tools (sensors) and the information processing power in today's smartphones, apps play a crucial role in collecting, collating and displaying this information to us in a way that makes sense and makes it useful to us. And more often than not, these apps are free or very inexpensive, symbolic of the new business models that complete the vying triumvirate of technology, medicine and stakeholder interests that will determine our ultimate success in bringing the potential to reality in the coming years.

Chapter 3:
Vital Signs

Paraphrasing the old saying that war is too important to be left to the military, medicine is too important to be left to doctors!

- Aristide Briand

Although we rely on doctors and other health care providers for our well-being, we are the ones who stand to gain the most from health and lose the most from ill-health. Never before in history have we had as much opportunity to influence our own personal future and simply knowing where to start is the first step to taking more control of our own destiny.

The clue is in the name - vital signs are our body's most important indicators of overall health and the first place that a medical professional will likely start in assessing our well-being. So it makes a lot of sense that these would be the starting point to give a baseline for anyone seeking to better understand their own body's key indicators.

While most modern cars come with a check engine light to alert the user to impending trouble, and virtually all gadgets have outward indicators of malfunctions, either in the form of flashing lights or beeps, humans are not so well equipped to clearly highlight any of the thousands of ailments that can afflict our bodies. And with the unfortunate fact that many potentially fatal conditions build up over long periods with little or no external or even internally palpable or perceptible symptoms, such an indicator would be most useful!

Understanding Vital Signs

The closest things to an outward warning light that humans have are probably our so-called vital signs. These are key indicators of a person's physical condition and if any of the readings is outside of a normal range, it can indicate serious issues. Most medical television dramas rely on hassled paramedics shouting these numbers to create a sense of urgency and tension when delivering a patient to ER doctors. While there is no universally agreed definition of vital signs, virtually all medical professionals agree on at least these four as crucial for determining the baseline current physical condition of a person:

- Heart Rate
- Blood Pressure
- Temperature
- Respiration

Depending on the circumstances, the next most important signs to check after these four may vary. For example, if a patient has been involved in a trauma or lost consciousness, the importance of pupil reaction is more urgent than it would be in a situation where they were complaining of an abdominal pain. In non-emergency settings, blood oxygen level is also a widely monitored sign and a good indicator of overall cardio-respiratory condition, while weight is increasingly considered a vital factor in determining a person's long-term health. Indeed, height, weight and the resultant Body Mass Index (BMI - body mass divided by the square of the body height expressed in kg/m^2) are considered in the US to be vital signs and globally are among the first personal measurements a general practitioner will note in a non-emergency context.

In this chapter, we will look at the array of technologies now available to closely monitor these vital signs and record/analyze them via a smartphone.

Home Help

Personal or home measurement of vital signs has been possible for quite some time. People with chronic heart problems have had domestic blood pressure monitors for many years and most households have at least a thermometer on hand to look for signs of fever.

But what has changed in the last couple of years is the availability, choice and cost of these devices but also their ability to store the results on a smartphone and onwards in an online repository. Coupled with the new tendency for people who are not yet displaying any symptoms or not yet diagnosed with any condition to take an interest in their health (the "worried well"), this ability to record and share the information makes the monitoring device immediately more useful. The fact that the app can attempt to interpret the results and present them in a wider context means that it's harder to ignore the indications. An app also can remind you that you haven't taken a reading or can advise you, based on a reading, to seek urgent help. The passive monitors of old that weren't connected to a smartphone relied too much on the patient taking the initiative to conduct the test, interpret the number and decide on a course of action. Recording the results was a hit-and-miss affair, prone to transcription errors or even willful manipulation.

Measuring multiple vital signs is now both possible and easy in the comfort of your own home and there is evidence that measuring vital signs in a non-clinical setting can give a more accurate reading than those taken in clinical settings due to "white coat syndrome" where people get stressed resulting in an elevated and non-typical cardiac reading. There is also of course the other side of the equation that home or amateur results may not be correctly recorded. In order to alleviate that risk, I would recommend that anyone monitoring their vital signs themselves uses only reputable equipment but, more importantly, compare the results periodically with those obtained by their healthcare professional with clinical grade devices.

While vital signs are important, it is also worth remembering that many serious conditions will not have an immediate impact on your vital signs, so you cannot take normal results on your vitals as a guarantee that nothing is wrong. It's also a good idea to decide in consultation with a medical professional on the frequency of measuring your vital signs so that intervals between measurements are appropriate.

Heart Rate Monitoring (HRM)

As the veritable engine of the body, the heart is the natural starting point for assessing physical condition. Your resting heart rate is a good indicator of overall fitness levels but your heart's well-being and that of the associated wider circulatory system will be heavily influenced by many of the factors discussed in this and the following chapters.

On average, the human heart beats around 40 million times a year. As always with averages, that number hides a multitude of variations and individual nuances. Your heart rate, or pulse, varies with age and fitness, as well as circumstances and medical condition. People on blood pressure medication may see a very low heart rate as well as controlled blood pressure. Aerobically fit people will typically have a lower resting heart rate than a less fit person - changes in your heart rate are an accurate means to understanding how your body is responding to exercise and the activities of daily life.

Many people I spoke to in researching this book were unaware that their heart rate varied naturally by as much as 50 % in the course of a day. This variability can be an indicator of stress as we shall see later. But while some variation is to be expected, anyone with unexplained variations in any vital sign should immediately seek professional advice.

Heart Rate Monitoring Benefits

While the constant approach to heart rate monitoring for decades, if not centuries, has been the finger on the wrist, more accurate recording tools for the heart's activities are now readily available - there is a range of sophisticated cardiac monitoring devices but the most basic is the heart rate monitor (HRM). For most healthy people, there may not be a huge medical benefit to heart rate monitoring. But it does provide a framework for exercise or at least an interesting insight into the invisible activity of your most vital organ, and a person may see their resting heart rate slow down after many months of exercise and physical improvement. But for some people who have high heart rate (tachycardia) or low heart rate (bradycardia) it may give a vital clue to seek timely medical guidance.

All Shapes and Sizes

As you'll see repeatedly throughout this book as a common theme, consumer technologies for HRM come in a variety of shapes and sizes, using different technologies to achieve the same ends, as single purpose devices or integrated with other features, and at a range of prices. Some heart rate monitors provide a snapshot of your current heart rate, while other solutions provide a continuous picture as you train, walk or sleep.

So if you've decided that you'd like to keep an eye on your heart rate, what are your options? These devices are for measuring either your active or resting heart rate. Measuring can be done via:

- Chest Strap
- Band/Watch
- Sensor built in to phone
- Adhesive Strip
- Phone case
- Phone & App
- Multi-purpose devices

Chest Strap

Until recently, most heart rate monitors came in the form of a small monitor that you strap to your chest. These devices, the size of a small stack of business cards, are strapped on to your chest and relay your heart rate to a watch or smartphone. While small enough to wear unobtrusively under clothes, these are most suited to people who need accurate, continuous monitoring such as when training. They are not best suited for quick checks of your heart rate as you need to apply the strap and monitor and then refer to the accompanying watch or smartphone app. These straps are typically available from about $50 or less. Popular models are available from fitness companies Garmin and Polar, among others.

Ampstrip

A new entrant in the heart rate monitoring arena is a product called the Amstrip. A good example of the new practice of crowdsourcing[1] funding for the development of new products, this 3.5" long heart rate monitor attaches on your torso much like a Band-Aid. This is slightly more convenient than strapping on a sensor, is rechargeable offering 7-10 days battery life, and works while swimming too. You simply apply a new adhesive strip to reuse the sensor. The clear focus of this product is on atheletes' training. However, I see it as the precursor of a new generation of sensors that you can attach to the body and I can envisage many other sensors following this form factor given the increased likelihood of patient compliance if the sensor is hassle free and comfortable to wear.

---

[1] Crowdsourcing refers to the use of web sites to collect funding directly from individuals to bring an unreleased product or idea to market without following traditional capital raising practices. Popular sites include Indiegogo.com and Kickstarter.com

Wrist-Based

While many chest strap monitors relay their data to a watch that is easily viewable while training, there has been a rapid growth in the number of devices that actually take the measurement from the wrist. Although there are several points around the body where heart rate can be measured, the wrist is one of the most accessible sites. The majority of wrist-worn heart rate trackers rely on optical sensors - they shine a light onto your wrist and measure the blood flowing through your capillaries. A more recent entrant into this sphere is the Jawbone Up 3 activity tracker that includes bioimpedance sensors to report on your resting heart rate via small electrical impulses. This has the advantage over optical solutions of requiring less battery power - a key consideration for designers of wearable devices. The Jawbone device reports your heart rate to the accompanying app which we'll see again later in the sections on activity, diet and sleep.

You can purchase dedicated continuous heart rate monitoring wrist devices or increasingly, the technology is being built in to watches. The majority of smartwatches can now tell you your heart rate - some without even pushing a button. If I say "OK Google, show me my heart rate", I don't even have to take my hands away from the keyboard and in about 10 seconds my Android Wear smartwatch reports that my heart rate is a satisfactory 75 beats per minute.

Optical sensors face a number of technical challenges when it comes to accuracy - they require you to keep very still to take a reading and skin pigmentation can be an obstacle to clear readings. In tests, some struggle to offer accurate results at very high heart rates, such as those seen during extreme physical exertion. However, most deliver results that are within +/- 10% of more definitive measurements. This is probably accurate enough to help you get a sense of your heart health and unexpected changes should be investigated urgently.

Built-In

Given that, for most healthy people, the value of frequent heart rate monitoring is relatively small, the thoughts of investing in a separate accessory for this task may seem excessive. But for those with even a curiosity, there are several solutions available that don't require an additional purchase or the need to wear a strap or attach any sensors.

With the Galaxy S5 model, Samsung introduced a built-in heart rate sensor, a first for a phone. Simply by opening the supplied S-Health App and placing your finger over the sensor below the camera on the rear of the device, you can measure your resting heart-rate. Obviously this can only be used to get a snapshot of your heart rate as it's not suitable to run and hold your fingertip steady over the sensor!

Having a built-in sensor has advantages - it removes the need for a person to take any proactive action to procure the ability to monitor. Even if people only use it to show off how their new phone is "cool", and while I'm sure many S5 and S6 phones go through their daily lives without ever being asked to monitor a heart rate, I'm equally sure that the inclusion has brought heart rate monitoring to people who would otherwise not have access to it.

Smartphone - Camera & App

For those who only have a passing interest in their health (as is often the case for people who are exhibiting no symptoms), checking your vital signs is, as we've said, a curiosity but hardly worthy of purchasing accessories. Given that relatively few phone models incorporate heart-rate sensors, the existence of apps that purport to measure your vital signs with no peripherals offer a chance for a huge number of smartphone owners to satisfy their curiosity and have some fun doing so. So what exactly do you do if you want to know your heart rate but don't have a top of the line Samsung phone and you don't want to buy an accessory?

There are two app-based approaches to measuring your heart rate - both use the increasingly sophisticated cameras found on today's smartphones. In the first example, there are several apps which work by having you place your finger over the rear camera lens on your phone and turning on the flashlight. The app then analyses the image in the camera and detects the changes in color caused by the blood flow as your heart beats. If that sounds far-fetched, there is solid science behind it - the rather impressively named Photoplethysmography - the same technology you'll find in virtually every hospital where it's used in dedicated pulse oximeter devices which measure blood oxygen saturation levels.

"Let me Look at You"

For the second app-only HRM option, the premise of the Philips Vital Signs app is quite amazing - simply look at the camera on the front of your phone and it will tell you your heart rate and your breathing rate. I must admit that I was hugely skeptical of these claims when I first came across this app. The only thing that probably prevented me from simply dismissing it as a fake and moving on was that it was produced by such a reputable name in medical equipment. Surely a worldwide leader in the supply of some of the most sophisticated sensors in the world to leading hospitals wouldn't waste its time and its reputation by producing something so inaccurate as to be useless? So I downloaded the app and tried it. It was one of those rare 'wow' moments that you get occasionally from technology. Here was a free app on my phone that without even touching me could tell my heart rate.

So how does it work? Simply download the app to your iPhone, open the app and look at the screen. Hold the phone steady and place your face in the square indicated on the screen. The camera on the front of the phone then analyses the minute changes in the color of your face caused by your heart beat. Imperceptible to the human eye, the camera on the phone is sensitive enough to see these changes and time their frequency.

As well as monitoring your heart rate, the app also reports your breathing rate, this time based on the up and down movement of your chest as you breathe. You can of course fool it by holding your breath but that doesn't really help!

Both the heart and breath results are plotted against a "normal" continuum. You have the option to store or share your results by email or social network. As with all the technologies discussed here, the app comes with a disclaimer that its results are for entertainment purposes only and not for medical diagnosis purposes. The app even offers a valentine mode that measures two people together. But don't blame me if you end up having a row because your partner doesn't set your heart racing ;). Without doubt, the Philips Vital Signs camera app is an innovative app that's enjoyable to use and perhaps the least invasive health monitoring technology I've come across.

I was skeptical of the accuracy you can expect from a phone re-purposed to a heart rate monitor, but it's increasingly advisable not to underestimate the sheer power of the sensors in these pocket devices we take for granted. It is scarcely credible what can be achieved with pocket-sized purpose-built accessories that work with smartphones, so it may seem even more unlikely that an app alone can monitor your heartbeat with any degree of accuracy - but that would be to underestimate the creative ways that people are now harnessing the computing and sensing power in modern smartphones.

Again, it's worth repeating that these are not medical grade devices, and while they may not be as accurate, you should be able to discern fluctuations in your vital signs that may signal a need for a medical assessment.

Multi-Purpose Devices

The dramatic rise to prominence of the smartphone has typified the emergence of multi-purpose devices in the modern era. Just as the computer fulfills many different tasks, an increasing number of devices that significantly extend the already impressive capabilities of smartphones have emerged. The falling cost and size of sensors means that most accessories aimed at health-conscious individuals can now offer multiple measurements.

A quick glance at the Appendix lists the devices I tried for heart rate monitoring reveals several devices that appear in other categories too. Given the relative simplicity of heart rate readings, it seems to be a favorite for manufacturers to include alongside the other attributes they are more focused on measuring. Here are just some of the examples of devices that offer HRM as one of their many readings - we'll look at some of these devices in more detail in later sections where they are described in line with their primary purpose:

- Withings Pulse - this tiny activity tracker also includes an optical sensor for heart rate monitoring.
- Alivecor - this personal ECG device clips on to the back of your phone and reports your heart rate while it focuses on more detailed heart activity analysis - more on that later
- Bathroom scales - there are several smart scales on the market now that include heat rate measurement with tiny electrical impulses as you stand on it. We'll talk more about advanced scales later in this chapter.

Headphones

Both LG and Jabra make headphones that monitor your heart rate. Again, this might sound like a strange combination of technologies but given that many athletes and joggers listen to music while running/training it makes a lot of sense. Much less hassle than strapping on and off a chest-based sensor, these devices look and work like normal headphones with the addition of a small sensor to monitor heart rate as you walk, cycle or run, with your heart rate reported back to your phone via Bluetooth as the phone sends the music to the earphones in the opposite direction. Recent apps can even vary the tempo of the music they send based on your activity level!

Heart Rate and Exercise

So there's no doubt that you have several options if you want to measure your heart rate. If you are interested in learning more about your heart rate and its influence on training, it's worth reading up on the topic of maximum heart rate. This is the maximum recommended rate during exercise. You can then target various heart rate zones - your heart rate elevation relative to its maximum recommended rate - each of which has a different impact on the outcome of your training for example in weight loss, stamina or post training recovery.

The Mayo Clinic provides the following guidance: The basic way to calculate your maximum heart rate is to subtract your age from 220. That means that if you're 45 years old, subtract 45 from 220 to get a maximum heart rate of 175. This is the maximum number of times your heart should beat per minute while you're exercising. For example, exercising at 60-70% of your maximum heart rate is the most effective for weight loss - Training in Zone 2 (in this example maintaining an active heart rate of up to 125) enhances endurance and the efficiency with which you use fat and carbohydrates as fuel. Some call this the "fat-burning zone" because this is the best zone to train in for those who wish to lose weight.

So why all this emphasis on heart rate measurement? As you'll being to appreciate when we continue to look at activity and diet and the massive challenge of weight control, quite aside from the insight into your cardiac well-being, knowing more about your heart rate is crucial in designing effective exercise plans. Also, an awareness of your heart rate can assist in ensuring you don't push yourself too hard too often. If you're short of breath, in pain or can't work out as long as you'd planned, your exercise intensity is probably higher than your fitness level allows.

Continuous heart rate feedback lets you know whether you are in your heart rate training zone for your specific fitness goal – whether that's fat-burning, aerobic conditioning, anaerobic threshold training, or general cardiovascular fitness. If you are not training and not concerned about a heart problem then you are unlikely to need continuous monitoring or expect to gain any actionable insights from it - for people in general good health, periodic measurement is usually fine.

For those looking at even more detail on their heart rate and training, some devices also include your Maximal oxygen uptake (VO$_2$ max) which is a measure of the maximum volume of oxygen that an athlete can use and is widely accepted as a strong measure of cardiovascular fitness and maximal aerobic power. It is measured in milliliters per kilogram of body weight per minute (ml/kg/min) and is estimated (from the devices discussed in this book) by the Microsoft Band and the LG Headphones, among others - based on your heart rate and the Rockport Walk Test Formula. So as not to risk alienating readers not that interested in training, I mention it here as an example of more detailed and actionable information available once you've started measuring your heart rate but I'll leave the more dedicated among you to look it up.

Blood Pressure

If heart rate is one of the easiest measures of our cardiac activity, it is the blood pressure that results from our heart pumping that has become perhaps the single most common and widely discussed vital sign measurement in the last couple of decades. As our understanding of the heart has improved, so too has our certainty that blood pressure is a hugely important indicator of well-being and a key influencer of cardiac outcomes. It's safe to say that everyone of us knows someone who has been diagnosed with high blood pressure and statistics show that about thirty-three percent of adults in the U.S. have high blood pressure. Globally, that number jumps to 40%, but many people with the condition remain unaware or go untreated because there are no real signs or symptoms for high blood pressure. Most of us know that blood pressure is an important measurement of heart health, but what exactly is it, and why does it matter?

Blood Pressure refers to the pressure exerted by your heart pumping, at the maximum and minimum points of its pulsing cycle. Typically quoted in two numbers, a person's blood pressure is usually expressed in terms of the systolic (the maximum pressure in the arteries when the heart contracts, squeezing freshly oxygenated blood into the arteries) over the diastolic (the minimum pressure in the arteries between heartbeats while the heart rests and refills between beats) pressure. So for example, an ideal blood pressure reading is generally agreed to be no higher than 120/80, measured in a unit of pressure known as mm/HG - millimeters of mercury. However, the risk of cardiovascular disease increases progressively above 115/75 mm Hg.

Blood pressure varies depending on situation, activity, and disease states. Various factors, such as age and sex, influence a person's blood pressure and variations in it. Systolic and diastolic arterial blood pressures are not static but undergo natural variations from one heartbeat to another and during the day. They also change in response to stress, nutritional factors, drugs, disease, exercise, and even momentarily from standing up. A well-known example of changed blood pressure is so called "white coat syndrome "- where, in up to 25% of patients, the blood pressure measurement in a hospital or clinic is higher than their typical blood pressure measured without the "stress" of a medical professional or clinical environment.

Why Is Blood Pressure Important?

Blood pressure directly affects the health of our blood vessels, the veins and arteries that pervade our bodies. Healthy blood vessels are robust and remarkably flexible, able to withstand the constant pressure of blood rushing throughout the body for decades. Over time however, chronic high blood pressure can cause damage to otherwise healthy blood vessels, and such damage puts us at risk for several severe health conditions like heart attacks, stroke, kidney failure and more.

Blood pressure that is pathologically high is called *hypertension* in medical circles. Chronic hypertension often goes undetected because of the absence of obvious symptoms and the fact that traditionally it was only screened for by doctors. Over time, high or low blood pressure can lead to and/or be indicative of bigger health problems, so these are important numbers to know.

While genetics play a significant role in your predisposition to elevated blood pressure, positively influencing your blood pressure has a number of well-documented factors that are within most people's control. Some factors that may cause high blood pressure include age, race, family history, overweight or obesity, physical inactivity, smoking, poor diet (think: too much sodium, too little potassium), stress, high alcohol consumption and certain other medical conditions, such as kidney disease, sleep apnea and hypothyroidism (an inactive thyroid gland).

Measuring Blood Pressure

So now that you're hopefully convinced of the importance of knowing and monitoring your blood pressure, it's time to look at the tools available to measure it, before we look in the following chapters in more detail at the exercise and diet tools available should you need to take action based on the blood pressure readings you discover.

As we've just seen, blood pressure fluctuates from minute to minute depending on factors like posture, hydration, activity level, the presence of stress or anxiety, and sleep. These moderate, short-term changes in blood pressure are normal and healthy. They're simply the body's way of making sure oxygenated blood gets to where it is needed. Since blood pressure varies frequently throughout the day, measurements intended to monitor changes over longer time frames should be taken at the same time of day and in the same circumstances to ensure that the readings are comparable and indicative of the underlying values.

Checking Blood Pressure was traditionally the preserve of doctors but a quick look for home blood pressure monitors on Amazon.com reveals no less than 1065 different models, ranging in price from a mere $15 to over $600. Clearly the personal BP market offers considerable choice and increasingly monitors are now linked to smartphones wirelessly to make it easier to record and analyze the data.

The technical term for a blood pressure monitor is a Sphygmomanometer and they have been a staple of doctor's surgeries in pretty much their current form since 1901. Although a quite fun word to say, most people probably just call it a blood pressure meter. These devices measure blood pressure through a cuff, usually attached to the upper left arm/bicep. Domestic monitors are largely electronic, with LCD displays so the user can easily see the reading. Although considered slightly less accurate, wrist-mounted meters are increasingly common due to their increased convenience and portability.

Wireless Blood Pressure Monitors (Cuff/Wrist)

A number of companies now produce blood pressure monitors and accompanying apps to ease the recording of blood pressure. A cuff device typically costing less than $100 is placed on the arm/wrist and communicates wirelessly with the user's smartphone via Bluetooth. The app associated with the smart blood pressure monitor is typically used to initiate the reading once the user has secured the cuff. Illustrations on the phone screen can assist in ensuring that the device is correctly positioned and gyroscope sensors can alert the app when the appropriate height is reached. The cuff is then inflated and the heart rhythm displayed on the phone's screen. After approx. 30 seconds, the cuff deflates and the systolic and diastolic readings are displayed, along with the interpretation of the reading on the scale of blood pressure from a recognized medical body. The app also shows the historic trends of previous measurements.

In a break with the long established tradition of cuff-style blood pressure monitors, there are now alternative technologies emerging that are less hassle to use to determine blood pressure. I've tried two such devices where their primary purpose isn't actually blood pressure measurement - it's just one of a number of features they offer. We'll have a look at one such hand-held device later in this chapter and one wrist-mounted one in a later chapter.

Action on Blood Pressure Information

If your domestic blood pressure reading is outside of normal ranges, you should consult a medical professional. But there are plenty of well-established lifestyle changes said to assist in the reduction of high blood pressure and many of these are supported by the technologies in the following chapters.

ECG

If you are interested in better understanding your heart health, there are options beyond just blood pressure and heart rate monitors. While every neighborhood doctor's surgery is equipped with such basic medical diagnosis devices, few have typically had the facility to carry out more advanced tests such as electrocardiograms, or ECGs.

An ECG is the process of recording the electrical activity of the heart - during each heartbeat, a healthy heart will have an orderly pattern of depolarization which gives rise to the characteristic ECG tracing. To the trained clinician, an ECG conveys a large amount of information about the structure of the heart and the function of its electrical conduction system. Among other things, an ECG can be used to measure the rate and rhythm of heartbeats, the size and position of the heart chambers, the presence of any damage to the heart's muscle cells or conduction system, the effects of cardiac drugs, and the functioning of implanted pacemakers.

Until recently, ECGs required wiring a patient up to a large machine in a clinic or hospital. But thanks to miniaturization, you can now have a comparable device that sticks to the back of your phone and performs a similar function - the AliveCor ECG is a one such device. It is a wafer thin small sensor that you stick or hold on the back of your phone which carries out an ECG reading in just 30 seconds just by placing your fingertips on it. Record an ECG of at least 30 seconds, and the device will determine right away when your ECG is normal. It also allows you to send it off to a cardiologist who will review the data and respond within hours (for a fee of $10). And, you can always share your ECG with your own physician for no additional charge. This kind of access to sophisticated cardiac diagnosis is a far cry from the agonizing delay waiting for an appointment with a cardiologist. At an $75 price point, this technology is easily within the reach of a GP who could use it to gain a preliminary diagnosis and fine tune their referral process.

When I first came across this device nearly two years ago, it was nearly £200 and twice the size it is today. But although it is fully FDA approved (unlike many quasi-medical devices as we'll discuss in the section on Regulation), the price has more than halved along with the reduction in its dimensions. Alongside telling you your heart rate and supplying a trace to a cardiologist for review, its software has recently been upgraded so that it can automatically detect atrial fibrillation (AF). AF, a leading cause of stroke, is the most common heart rhythm disturbance. It affects over 140 million people worldwide, but the good news is that 3 out of 4 strokes can be prevented if detected and treated. The makers of this accessory report that they are already receiving over 10,000 readings per day, so clearly there are a lot of early adopters out there monitoring their heart health.

The AliveCor accessory makes use of the app/notification abilities of your smartphone by popping up reminders when you are due to conduct another ECG, but also provides a daily diary to record any drugs you are taking so that you can look to correlate any heart irregularities with missed doses.

Blood

Blood plays a critical role circulating in our body distributing essential substances and nutrients, such as sugar, oxygen, and hormones to our cells, and carrying waste away from those cells, as well as providing vital temperature regulation and infection-fighting services to our body. We rarely interact with our own blood, leaving the approximately 5 liters of fluid to silently go about its vibrant business.

From outside the body, we can quickly analyze the blood stream to determine its oxygen content (SpO_2), while anyone who has or knows someone who has diabetes will be well familiar with the ritual of testing glucose content. Deeper investigation than those usually involve the extraction and analysis of larger quantities of blood, but even this age old tradition is now evolving rapidly.

Blood Oxygen/Saturation

The human body requires and regulates a very precise and specific balance of oxygen in the blood. Hemoglobin is the protein in blood that carries oxygen and measuring oxygen saturation involves identifying how much of the available hemoglobin is loaded with oxygen. Normal blood oxygen saturation (sat) levels are considered to be between 95-100 percent of the available oxygen carrying capacity, though they may be lower at high altitudes. Having a low level of oxygen in your blood is known as hypoxemia and is usually a sign of respiratory problems or anemia which should be investigated.

Checking your blood oxygen levels at one time required a blood test and laboratory analysis, but now is a quick, non-invasive and totally painless task. In a process similar to the optical heart rate monitoring techniques discussed earlier, devices checking for blood oxygenation pass two wavelengths of light through the body part (usually a fingertip) to a photodetector. It measures the changing absorbance at each of the wavelengths, allowing it to determine the absorbances due to the pulsing arterial blood. If you're particularly interested in better understanding this magic, there's a very detailed yet understandable explanation of photoplethysmogrpahy and pulse oximetry available here: http://www.howequipmentworks.com/pulse_oximeter/

Blood Oxygen Measurement

When it comes to personal devices to check your oxygen saturation, you have several choices:

Dedicated Pulse Oximeter - these devices' primary purpose is the measurement of blood oxygen levels and typically clip on to the end of the finger, perhaps best described as a "clothes peg". Most devices of this type also monitor the heart rate. Wireless models report the blood oxygen level to the associated app when the phone is available but are capable of storing multiple readings internally. The iHealth device also reports the Perfusion Index (PI) which is a relative assessment of pulse strength at the measurement point.

The Samsung Galaxy S5 (which we noted earlier introduced a built in heart rate monitor), is also capable of recording blood oxygen levels using the same procedure of placing your finger over the sensor below the camera on the rear of the phone. Similarly, the Withings Pulse activity meter that includes a heart rate monitor simultaneously reports your blood oxygen levels. The Scanadu Scout multi-purpose device we'll cover in more detail later in this chapter also monitors SpO2 among its other metrics.

Blood Glucose

About 30 million people in the US (nearly 1 in ten) are believed to be suffering from diabetes (either diagnosed or not) and with alarming increases in the levels of pre-diabetes, domestic blood glucometers are already a well-established niche device. Just as with blood pressure monitors discussed earlier, these home and portable devices have existed for years. But the addition of smartphone recording and communication capabilities mean that it is now easier than ever to record, analyze and directly distribute results to doctors.

Testing for glucose is still a marginally invasive procedure - you use a small lancet to extract a drop of blood, place it on a test strip and put the test strip into a small reader device, usually about the size of a deck of playing cards. Recent models are wireless and use Bluetooth to sync the glucose result to the patient's phone where it joins all historical readings on handy trend graphs. The patient can also note their recent meal time (as this impacts readings) to help improve accuracy over old fashioned paper diaries.

Examples of mobile-enhanced readers include the iHealth Glucometer which comes in a basic model you have to plug in to your phone and in a Bluetooth variant that has an LED display on the device itself and wirelessly transmits historic data to the app. Vendors such as Integrity Applications are working with the FDA to get a fully non-invasive glucometer (in the form of an ear-clip) approved, along with an accompanying app.

Weight/Body Mass Index (BMI)

Although not always seen as a vital sign, weight is a hugely important measure of health and well-being, and is something that people are generally very familiar with measuring, even if all too often they don't like the result. Bathroom scales are a long time and even detested fixture in many houses. More recently, the emphasis has shifted from absolute weight measurement to BMI to give a relativity to the weight reading based on the gender and height of the person. While the exact merits of BMI are hotly debated in some circles, there is near total medical agreement that maintaining a suitable weight for an individual is one of the most important health factors for long term well-being and minimization of risk.

Leaving aside the metabolism (the biochemical process by which your body converts what you eat and drink into energy) and microbiota (the micro-organisms that live in your gut) differences between people and the impacts of some weight-impacting diseases, it's fair to say that for most people, their mass is determined to a significant extent by a combination of food intake and exercise.

The humble weighing scales has evolved beyond recognition in recent years. While it remains a flat box you stand on, your weight is now only one of a myriad of readings it can deliver, as imperceptible tiny electrical pulses enable these devices to read much more than a simple weight level - just remember to take off your socks or it can't work! As I stand on my Withings Body Analyzer (they don't even call it a scales anymore!), I can watch the large LCD display tell me my weight, my BMI, my body fat percentage and my heart rate before it continues to tell me the CO_2 level and temperature in the room, culminating in its grand finale of a display of today's weather forecast so I can dress appropriately! It then seamlessly provides all that information to a cloud backup service and onwards to my phone over WiFi so that it's all recorded, graphed and analyzed. Modern scales can even identify which different family member is standing on it and record each person's details individually.

Another model, the iHealth Core scale, now offers an almost overwhelming amount of detail for some, but the more granular breakdown of your overall weight may give real focus to your efforts to improve your body composition. Among its detailed readings are Body Fat and Body Water percentages, Lean Mass, Muscle Mass and Bone Mass in Kg, as well as your Visceral Fat Rating. All of this is done in a couple of seconds as you stand on the scales and fed back to your phone where you can clearly see any trends, and hopefully positive changes in any of the values you're targeting.

Some of these metrics it measures include:

- Body Fat % - the amount of body fat as a proportion of your body weight
- Bone Mass – the amount of bone material (calcium & minerals) in your body
- Muscle Mass – the weight of muscle in your body (including skeletal and other muscles)
- Body Water % - the total amount of fluid in your body as a % of your total weight
- Visceral Fat Rating – the fat level in your internal abdominal cavity

Remember that losing too much weight or the wrong kind of weight may have harmful effects on your well-being so this extra information can guide you and your healthcare professional to make more informed decisions.

Temperature

Thermometers have seen quite a degree of technological advancement in recent years from the mercury shaft in a glass tube that was placed under my tongue as a child to digital devices that report precise readings on easily-read numerical screens following the insertion of a sensor into the ear.

But the next logical stage in the development of this technology is to record the data on your smartphone, where it can be logged, graphed and recalled along with all your other vital sign data. And so you can now easily buy a smart thermometer such as the Kinsa – which relays the temperature under your tongue straight to your smartphone or you can even get adhesive patches such as TempTraq which relays your temperature to a phone continuously for 24 hours. These continuously reading devices have the advantage of enabling you to monitor for example an infant's temperature without having to disturb the child.

Respiration

Auscultation, the technical term for listening to the sound of the heart and lungs, usually with a stethoscope, has been the mainstay of the physical examination since the invention of the stethoscope way back in 1815. Until now, auscultation has required the presence of a physician but a digital stethoscope from a company called Clinicloud uses a smartphone app to guide users through the proper use of the device. Users can upload the chest sounds to a doctor for a professional opinion, along with the patient's temperature using the digital thermometer supplied in the $129 home health kit.

Aside from the Philips Vital signs app above, there are relatively few general purpose breathing-related devices for consumers. They are usually only necessary in cases where the patient has chronic symptoms but for people who are managing chronic conditions such as Asthma, Cystic Fibrosis (CF) or Chronic Obstructive Pulmonary Disease (COPD), then Spirometers are available that report your breathing power to an app, in place of more old fashioned devices and paper diaries.

Taking a different angle on respiration, where the focus is on the rate rather than the quality of the breath, the Spire wearable is a small clip-on device you wear on your belt that measures your breathing rate and deduces whether you are calm, focused or tense. The app can notify you and suggest a relaxation exercise if you are tense for more than a few minutes. I have noticed that although I wasn't aware of any tension, it does seem to highlight that I'm tense at times where I can trace back to being under pressure or involved in a difficult activity.

Slightly further in the future, there's an app called ResApp under development in the University of Queensland in Australia. Although only at proof of concept stage at time of writing, this app "listens" to your cough and determines if you might have pneumonia. Using the microphone on your smartphone and signal-processing algorithms, in tests it has diagnosed pneumonia and asthma with 90 percent accuracy.

Medical Science Fiction

I'm keen that each of the technologies presented in this book has a scientific beneficial medical basis and doesn't represent technology for technology's sake.

While much science fiction tends to focus on the imagined evolution of space travel, the existence of other lifeforms and new weapons like lasers, blasters and disruptors, the genre often also predicts dramatic advances in medical technologies. A prominent innovation portrayed in Star Trek as early as 1966 was the tricorder – a medical diagnosis device that you could point at someone and get a medical evaluation of them. While a fully-fledged medical tricorder remains some time away from coming to reality, there is definite progress in that direction. Funded by the X Prize Foundation and Qualcomm, there is a $10 million dollar prize fund for the first company or team to create a working tricorder. Although the prize requires the diagnosis of over a dozen conditions, you can already purchase devices that can measure a smaller number of signs:

- The first device of its kind to be available is the Scanadu Scout. This small handheld device about the size of a hockey puck can measure your temperature, heart rate, blood oxygen level and even blood pressure simply from touching it to your temple for just 30 seconds. It reports its findings back to your smartphone over bluetooth.

- Kito Azoi – this phone case includes heart rate sensors without adding significant bulk to your phone along with temperature, blood pressure, respiration and blood oxygen levels. Although not yet available at time of writing, this device promises to offer a one-stop-shop for easy vitals measurement. Ease of use is a crucial requirement for any of these technologies to catch on and simply holding this device is sufficient to take multiple readings.

It doesn't take much imagination to think of the benefits of such a method of vital sign checking in the future being employed in a hospital setting – a quick scan of the patient without the need for thermometers, blood pressure meter (sphygmomanometer) and assorted other devices. And the results could be added automatically and wirelessly to a patient's electronic chart. And it could be administered easily in a waiting room.

Advanced Investigations

After vital signs, you start to move into the limits of what you can determine from the outside. Moving any further has previously required invasive procedures, visits to clinics and lab results. Now we're entering an era of mineral tests at home, as well as urine analysis outside of medical facilities.

The era of reliance on doctors and laboratories for access to our inner workings is coming to an end. We may still rely on them for interpretation of non-routine results, but soon the analysis will likely be a combined effort between a doctor and a supercomputer, a combination that has proven to be significantly more effective than either in isolation.

Alongside the multitude of metrics that we've discussed that can be tracked non-invasively from outside the body, the insights that will become available via self-administered samples will skyrocket. The makers of the Scanadu Scout device have announced that their next product will be a home urine analysis kit for levels of glucose, protein, leukocytes, nitrites, blood, bilirubin, urobilinogen, microalbumin, creatinine, ketone, specific gravity, and pH in urine. The Scanadu app will guide users through the test procedure, process and store the test results (for trending over time), and explain them, including highlighting any readings that would trigger advice to see a medical professional. Already available in India, a solution from uChek enables smartphones to read sample sticks, compare them against expected readings and carry out tests not normally available outside clinics.

Another product on the short term horizon is the Cue. This mini home "laboratory" allows you to collect small samples from your body and analyse them for 5 molecules via either blood droplet: inflammation, vitamin D, fertility, or other samples influenza (nostril sample), and testosterone (saliva sample).

Blood Tests of the (near) Future

"I deeply believe it has to be a basic human right for every body to have access to the kind of testing infrastructure that can tell you about these conditions in time for you to do something about it"

- Elizabeth Holmes, CEO, Theranos

The vast majority of people will have blood tests at some point in their lives - and modern laboratory analysis can perform tests that analyze and identify literally hundreds of conditions based on the chemical composition of your blood. Aside from checking your blood type, virtually every hospital admission includes a blood panel - a standard set of tests. The most common of these is the Complete Blood Count (CBC) which is done to monitor overall health, to screen for some diseases, to confirm a diagnosis of some medical conditions, to monitor an existing medical condition, and to monitor changes in the body caused by medication.

While it's hard to rival a laboratory blood test for the discovery of what's going on in virtually all parts of your body, there are exciting advances in the field of blood tests that provide hope that these relatively invasive tests will become both less invasive and more available. Although not yet the purview of smartphones, I don't doubt that fully capable home laboratories will soon be available for those interested, and all but the smallest clinics/doctor's practices will have diagnostic capabilities that were only recently in reach of only the largest hospitals and dedicated laboratories.

This is not some fanciful ambition - because of new testing methods developed by startup Theranos (founded by Elizabeth Holmes, now the youngest self-made female billionaire in the US), a few drops of blood can now yield results that previously required a full vial. Her company can run hundreds of tests on a drop of blood far more quickly than could be done with whole vials in the past — and it costs a lot less. Most results are available in about four hours and each test costs less than 50% of standard Medicare and Medicaid reimbursement rates. If those two programs were to perform all blood tests at those prices, Theranos-based testing would save $202 billion over the next decade.

While Theranos testing is currently rolling out via Walgreens pharmacies in the US, history suggests that the technology involved will be miniaturized further and in the not too distant future end up closer to the consumer. Already, Theranos have demonstrated their consumer-savvy nature by creating an app for iPhone and Android to schedule tests, find local participating pharmacies and even view/track your results. Some of the Theranos tests have just received FDA clearance so it is a safe bet that the laboratory-based blood testing industry is facing a disruptive wave technologically impossible in the past.

Beyond improved access to the kinds of blood testing we're largely familiar with, slightly further ahead for most consumers, a product called MinION promises a portable DNA measurement future - already at less than $1,000 and the size of a USB stick, this type of device may one day enable personal genetic testing on demand in your own home.

Diagnostics: Beyond Vital Signs

Measuring a human's well-being beyond these vital signs generally involves either the category of technologies known collectively as Imaging (scans such as X-Ray, Ultrasound, CT, PET or MRI) or more invasive tests including more complex blood tests or the investigative use of scopes. People who are a little squeamish will be glad to know we won't be discussing such invasive tests in significant depth here. But it is important to highlight that although these areas are currently largely outside the remit of this book, I fully expect that a future updated edition would devote considerable space to these topics. For now, we'll just briefly summarize the direction that these technologies are evolving and you should be able to imagine quite easily how these too will challenge established practices.

Imaging departments today typically occupy an entire wing or floor of a hospital housing large, expensive machines that produce astonishingly detailed views of the internals of the human body. Anyone who has been in a current generation MRI machine will know that they are currently far from portable. But as you read this book and consider the progress made over recent years in miniaturizing technology, you won't be surprised to learn that there are several examples of imaging technology being made more widely available through size and cost reductions.

In the interests of making this volume as immediately practical as possible, I will leave further discussion on the mobilization and democratization of these technologies for another time as I expect we are still a few years away from high street availability of miniature ultrasound or MRI scanners. But such devices will come - first moving from hospitals to local primary care centers and then perhaps to pharmacies and eventually to interested individuals.

Vitals Summary

Vitals signs are essential in almost every setting of care. They are as close to a 'North Star' in healthcare as it gets, and are relatively noninvasive and low cost. No doctor would enter a clinical scenario without them. When you are in hospital, your vital signs are routinely monitored every few hours, or even continuously. Outside of this, we tend to pay scant attention to them.

Given our reliance on indicators across so many areas of life, it's strange we don't take more notice of our vital signs. Much of the tracking explained in the following chapters has the ultimate aim of enabling us to ensure that our vital signs remain within healthy ranges for as long as possible.

Chapter 4:
Activity Trackers

Activity trackers are already established as one of the best known categories of personal well-being technologies. Not only have they existed for quite some time in the form of simple step-measuring pedometers, but they provide one of the most widely relevant measurements with simple to understand outputs that don't require medical interpretation. They have also been one of the first existing product areas to be given a new lease of life with the addition of the mobile industry's attention, as well as product promotion from large brands, such as Nike. Nowadays you'll find a dazzling array of mobile-connected options in high street stores, not just sports stockists.

In this section, we'll look at why you would want to track your activity, the levels of activity that are recommended and then we'll look at the various types of activity trackers on the market, from those built-in to some phones to both multi-purpose and specialized accessories.

Is Activity Really That Important?

Regular physical activity is one of the most important things you can do for your health. According to the Centers for Disease Control and Prevention (CDC) in the US, it can help:

* Control your weight
* Reduce your risk of cardiovascular disease
* Reduce your risk for type 2 diabetes and metabolic syndrome
* Reduce your risk of some cancers
* Strengthen your bones and muscles
* Improve your mental health and mood
* Improve your ability to do daily activities and prevent falls, if you're an older adult
* Increase your chances of living longer

Scientific research consistently emphasizes the health benefits of physical activity, and its ability to decrease the risk of massive killers - heart disease and diabetes. The World Health Organization (WHO) estimates that 27% of diabetes cases and 30% of all coronary diseases could be avoided with regular physical activity. Inactivity is one of the five main causes of mortality worldwide, along with: high blood pressure, tobacco use, hyperglycemia, and overweight and obesity.

A recent 12-year study of over 300,000 people published in the American Journal of Clinical Nutrition found that twice as many deaths were connected with lack of physical activity compared to obesity. Using the most recent available data on deaths in Europe the researchers estimate that 337,000 of the 9.2 million deaths amongst European men and women were attributable to obesity (classed as a Body Mass Index - BMI - greater than 30): however, double this number of deaths (676,000) could be attributed to physical inactivity. And while we'll tackle obesity in the next chapter, it's worth noting that more people are inactive than obese with 23 per cent of people in Ireland classified as obese but more than 50 per cent inactive.

The scientific definition of physical activity is any movement produced by muscular contractions that leads to an energy expenditure higher than the resting expenditure. Physical activity does not necessarily mean playing a sport, or completing an intense workout. Simply walking for 30 minutes a day, for example, is considered a regular physical activity proven to yield numerous health benefits. 30 minutes a day of moderate-intensity activity (such as a brisk walk) is linked to a 30% decrease in the risk of early mortality. Physical activity also has immense mental health benefits. In fact, studies have shown that physical activity has positive effects in preventing and treating depression.

The easiest way to start using technology to support a healthier lifestyle is probably to acquire an activity tracker. Today, the pedometer, imagined 400 years ago by Leonardo Da Vinci and first developed in 1965, has evolved far beyond a "step counter" and into a suite of full-service health tracking devices. The majority of wearable health devices are focused on activity tracking, though with some devices now supporting over 30 different measurements, companies making heart rate, blood pressure, glucose, and temperature devices are pushing trackers into the sphere of multi-purpose diagnostic solutions.

Move it and Lose it

Most people know that exercise is good for them, and they also know that they probably don't get enough every day. But if you ask people how much exercise they actually get versus how much they should get, you will likely find exact answers few and far between. You will also find people have very different understandings of what constitutes exercise. While some think that only going to the gym to work out or jogging count, others think rather optimistically that walking from their desk to the canteen on the floor below and back is sufficient.

The World Health Organization recommends that you should move 10,000 steps a day. That equates to roughly 90 minutes of walking, or a rather daunting 5 miles a day. And before you get excited that you walk 5 miles a day and can then pig out, it actually only represents an additional 20% calories on top of your daily allowance. Or to put a product on it, not even a King Size Mars bar.

But exercising is not all about weight management - it has two main benefits; while it burns calories which can help you lose weight, or make room for some extra treats, it also increases your fitness levels with benefits for cardiovascular, pulmonary (lung) and other areas. Getting sufficient exercise has proven positives for reducing risk of diabetes and strokes among other nasty diseases.

Of course, 10,000 steps is only a recommendation and a goal rather than an absolute necessity. There is nothing to prove that someone who gets 10,000 steps a day is dramatically healthier than someone who gets 9,000. What's important is that the human body does need a certain, not insignificant, amount of exercise to stay in shape. I would encourage people to understand how much exercise they are actually getting on a daily basis (you may be surprised either way about how much that is) and then resolve to increase it by as much as is practical. If all you can manage in the day is 7,000 and that's an improvement on where you are today, then set your target at 7,000 and go for it before you start over-obsessing on reaching 10,000.

The upside is that reaching that level of activity is good for your well-being, and also earns you a little latitude on your diet (more on diet in the next Chapter).

But I Don't Have Time!

One of the most frequent barriers to getting sufficient exercise is perceived lack of time. People often believe they don't have time to devote to exercise. Without getting into a philosophical debate about how investing time into your health now can mean you have more time to live, I'll focus on the day-to-day challenge of making time for exercise and we'll talk more about motivation later.

Virtually everybody gets some exercise during the day, so the good news is that you're unlikely to be starting from zero and trying to find time to rack up the entire 10,000 steps. When I first started counting my steps, I was surprised to find that I usually acquired about 2,000 steps a day in the course of my apparently sedentary office job. So that was a bonus - 20% of the day's target in the course of going to and from meetings, nipping across the road for a sandwich at lunchtime and general movement. Switching from using the lift to the stairs added another 500 steps a day (our office at the time was only 4 stories high).

But while an average office day may yield 2,000 steps, getting towards 10,000 undoubtedly takes a lot of effort, unless you have a more active job. People with active jobs have a steps advantage over desk-based professions. You rarely see overweight construction workers, for good reason. Identifying ways to include more activity in your day will be different for different people but it's worth considering ways to include more exercise in your daily routine. While the most obvious is perhaps to dedicate time to getting exercise by visiting a gym, going for a run/cycle/swim or similar dedicated approach, there are several other things you can do that might be easier to integrate into your day and require no memberships:

- Get off the bus/train a stop or two early and walk to the office or home
- Park your car further away from your destination and walk the rest of the way
- Go for a walk before/after work or at lunchtime

If you live in a city covered by CityMapper, this navigation and transit app will helpfully tell you not only the time/distance between two points, but also the calories you can expect to burn by choosing to walk or cycle instead of using the underground, bus or car.

Finding the time for activity in your lifestyle is going to be hard in most cases. But if you increase the intensity, you can decrease the amount of time you need. So the 90 minutes of walking mentioned above equates to more like 30 minutes of jogging. If you are very time-poor, you may not have the luxury of creating an extra hour in the day to walk so you'll have to look at other ways to integrate more exercise into your existing routine. While knowing how many steps you are getting vs how many you should get is useful, finding time is a genuine consideration. Without a plan, you're not going to find it easy to meet that rather challenging goal. If you really can't find time to add more exercise into your day, the best I can suggest is that you walk faster when you do have time to walk - and there are activity trackers that can specifically help you with that if that's what you need.

It's not all doom and gloom about fitting activity into your daily routine. Depending on your lifestyle, it may be easy or hard to make time, but knowing the scale of the challenge is a big step forward (pun intended) and to do this you need to know how much or how little of the daily target you already typically achieve.

I take great encouragement from the fact that small changes can make a big difference. The inactivity alert on your phone, smartwatch or tracker that prompts you to move after too many minutes of inactivity. Taking the stairs instead of the lift. Getting off the bus a couple of stops early. If you do have a desk job, it's all too easy to sit there and not move for hours on end. A reminder - take a walk to the water cooler - it's good for you to get steps, it's good for you to drink water and who knows who you might meet there for one of those (in)famous water cooler conversations.

Another insight I personally gained was that while my weekday activity level was well under control when I started walking to work instead of getting the bus, my app highlighted that without the workday routine, my weekend activity levels were shockingly low. While most of us like to take it easy at the weekend, it's also the time when we're most likely to overindulge on food, so all the more important to keep up any good exercise habits you have from during the week.

For those who can find the time, but regard exercise as boring, I highly recommend trying either music or audiobooks as a companion if you can't persuade someone to join you in your healthy choices. Not surprisingly given the theme of this book, this is an area where I believe apps can provide simple access to a wealth of content. Personally, my Spotify and Audible subscriptions mean that I have no shortage of company, entertainment and information when out for a walk if I don't fancy listening to my own thoughts. In fact, I would say that this multi-tasking has been a surprising additional benefit for me of creating time to go for walks. I have listened to more books in the last 12 months than I had read in the last 12 years, and now see time spent walking as additional time I have created to read rather than time lost to "just" exercising. And while we'll talk about brain exercise in a later chapter, research studies show that music and audiobooks provide clinically significant cognitive stimulation.

Another product that could prove useful and efficient as you exercise is a battery called "Ampy". This device which, is about the size of a deck of cards and about the same weight as an average smartphone, uses your motion to charge its battery. So by strapping this device on your belt or your arm while you walk or exercise, you can earn an hour of charge for your phone for each hour of activity. Then just connect your phone to the Ampy for an all-important battery top-up.

Measuring In All Shapes And Sizes

So if you're convinced that you should start measuring your steps in order to understand how many you get and how many more you need, where do you start? A simple search for fitness trackers on Amazon now returns over 2,000 hits, and that doesn't include trackers built in to phones and other devices.

In this section, I'm going to describe some of the key attributes you might consider when choosing an activity tracker but at the risk of jumping to the conclusion, I'm not going to recommend a specific product. I'll outline considerations I think you may find useful in picking out one that suits your needs, but the mere fact you're interested in acquiring one means you can't go too far wrong. Because it's worth saying it now, and I'll doubtless say it again in later chapters - this is not about the technology itself….what's important is how it can help identify and enable changes to your behavior to ultimately move you towards a better outcome for you and your health.

Fitness accessories will compete for your attention on aesthetics, phone compatibility, app experience, advanced functionality, or price point. Sure, there are features that might make a particular device more suitable for you than another one, but ultimately, the fact that you're using a gadget to inform your health and lifestyle choices should matter more than the selection you make. What I hope to do here is point out various features that might make such a device a better fit in your lifestyle and therefore something you are more likely to retain and get more benefit from.

As I said at the start of this section, activity tracking isn't really new. Dedicated pedometers that you clip on to your belt have been around for quite a few years. These simple devices simply display the day's steps on a small LCD screen. While sufficient for the job, they were not connected devices - the didn't report the trends to your phone. On the plus side though of their simplicity, they didn't typically need to be charged every few days! Some of the products available actually fit in multiple categories - e.g. some are clip-on or wrist mounted, while others that feature a heart rate monitor and blood oxygen level could have been discussed in the previous chapter. For simplicity's sake, I've tried to discuss relevant products under the heading where I think they best fit, with some consideration for their manufacturer's primary market positioning of them, as I think it fairest to mention products in their intended context.

So what has changed that has made pedometers seem old fashioned and activity trackers one of the hot new gadgets? Well, the fundamental technology is largely the same but the size/shape of the pedometer has evolved. The biggest change, though, is that the device now communicates with your phone (usually over Bluetooth) so you can record, analyze and even share your progress. Early models required to be plugged in to your phone or PC to see your results, which is not ideal when you want a quick update during the day on your progress. Advances in wireless technologies, particularly the development of a new low-power, short-range variant of Bluetooth (Version 4, also known as Bluetooth Smart, Bluetooth Low Energy or BLE) now means trackers can communicate with your phone several times an hour and still offer a battery life measured in weeks rather than days. And most of these have replaced the earlier cumbersome pairing rituals that dogged early implementations of Bluetooth technologies.

Apart from the advances made possible by wireless communication, the sophistication of the sensors now available is something that was unimaginable just a few years ago. The range of activity trackers available is not just about the size/shape and color but different solutions hide a dazzling array of features that will appeal to a variety of people depending on what level of detail they will find useful to enable and motivate them in their quest for a healthier lifestyle. Simple step counters are the dominant product in this category. These just count the number of steps you take and report it back to an app on your phone. But for those interesting in knowing more, you can choose from an array of more capable gadgets that add elevation, distance, cadence, degree of joint movement and even g-force impact of your feet with the ground. While this may seem like overkill if all you want to do is get closer to 10,000 steps a day, for those who are training or perhaps investigating knee pain, knowing that you're experiencing higher than average impact on one foot may be a very useful insight.

With a Flick of Your Wrist....

The leading fitness trackers are currently wrist-worn devices. These small bracelets are meant to unobtrusively monitor your movement throughout the day as you go about your business and with the majority of them being splash-proof if not fully waterproof, you can wear them in the shower, ensuring you don't miss out on any of your day's movement, however small. Most models offer at least a week's battery life and almost all come in a range of sizes and colors to suit different arm sizes and tastes. Sensors called accelerometers detect motion and decipher if the motion relates to a step or not. So as I sit here and type, the band on my wrist knows that I am not getting exercise. But as soon as I stand up and walk, it begins to register that movement and increase my daily step count. It can be fooled - so if I shake my arm around in a certain way, it does register that as a step, even though I'm still sat here, just looking a little silly waving my arm about. I suppose you could even argue that while not technically a step, my chair-obics (sounds a more legitimate name than "mad arm waving") are in fact burning up (very small) amounts of calories.

People who notice the little gadget on my wrist often ask me if the wristband is uncomfortable. I have to say I find it completely comfortable and as natural as wearing a watch - it's something you very quickly forget about. I've grown so accustomed to wearing it that I notice its absence when I have to take it off to charge - which luckily is only for a couple of hours every week or so.

The best known consumer examples in the step counting category are the Fitbit range and the Jawbone Up devices, as well as products from more athlete-focused Garmin and Polar. The Vivofit from Garmin trades continuous syncing and display quality for year-long battery life while the Polar Loop integrates with other Polar devices such as their Heart Rate Monitors. Sony and Samsung produce companion devices for smartphones. The Nike Fuelband was also a popular device in this arena, but Nike have recently stopped producing it as they move to a more app-led approach, letting others build the hardware.

Smartwatches avoid some of the obvious visibility of dedicated tracking wristbands. As most people wear a watch, it is only the more observant who may notice the type of watch and its purpose beyond telling the time. For those who want to avoid a techy smartwatch look, Withings make the Activite line - analog watches with a built in activity sweep arm and a battery life of over 6 months - these look like perfectly conventional watches. And while they still synchronize data back to an app on your phone, they do so without the obvious digital nature of leading smart watches such as Apple Watch or Android Wear models. Habitual watch wearers will find most of their steps will be counted without the need to don an additional piece of technology. But with most smartwatches requiring daily charging, they lack the wear and forget approach you can have for a week or more with the activity wristbands.

Wrist trackers generally have the following characteristics:

- Good accuracy
- Additional features such as heart rate
- Not always aesthetically attractive
- Battery life up to two weeks (for rechargeable, or 6 months for watch-cell powered)
- Always on you - even in the shower or for sleep
- independent of phone charge state

- can be hidden subtly under a sleeve
- have to come off to charge
- prone to knocks
- may be uncomfortable
- may be distracting - eg vibrations for messages/flashing lights

Clip It On

The next most common form factor for activity trackers is clip-on devices. Slightly confusingly, these often come with wrist straps so you can wear them on your wrist, but they are primarily sold as gadgets you can clip on or wear, depending on what activity you're tracking or perhaps just what you are wearing.

The leading clip-on devices are produced by Jawbone (Up Move), Misfit (Flash, Shine) and Withings (Pulse Ox). The obvious advantage of clip-on over wrist-worn is that you can be totally discreet with the former. Rather than proclaiming your step-measuring interest via your wrist, you can clip these trackers onto your belt or other suitable location, safely out of view. Just be careful where you secure it if you pick one that is magnetically attached - if you come across a tracker stuck to the center door exit pole on a number 91 London bus, I'd like it back!

While the discretion of clip-ons is appealing, the one drawback to keep in mind with them is that you do have to remember to clip them on and off your clothes (though some will actually survive a trip in the washing machine - and while it's not recommended I can vouch for the fact it can happen, but I suggest you be honest and not count the "steps" from its 90 minutes of tumbling and spinning) and clip-ons are not ideal for anyone who needs those few steps to and from the shower to reach the target - wrist worn are more suitable for sleep and they catch those few extra steps around the house before you put on your clothes and attach your clip-on model.

Another advantage of the clip on model is that many have a replaceable coin/watch battery rather than a rechargeable cell built in. This means that battery life is measured in months rather than days or weeks. For people who are less interested and want minimal hassle, these provide a low-interaction model that is very appealing. Most include a setting in the app so the sensor knows where on the body it's clipped to assist its algorithm's accuracy.

Clip-on characteristics:

- discrete - can clip anywhere
- you need to remember to clip them on
- risk of loss if you forget to take them off clothes at the end of the day
- great flexibility of where you wear it
- some manufacturers have specially designed socks and t-shirts with little pouches
- more discrete than wrist, though can choose wrist with supplied or optional straps

Build It In

For people who don't want any additional device beyond what they currently use but who do want to track their activity, two options have emerged more recently other than dedicated wrist bands or clip on pedometers - you can now find step tracking sensors in most smart watches and even in several high-end phones. The pros and cons of each of these approaches closely mirrors those of dedicated wrist and clip on devices but without the need to remember or charge additional gadgets.

The inclusion of step tracking sensors within phones themselves is an interesting development. This means you can track your steps just by carrying your phone with you. And with smartphones such an integral part of everyday life for so many people, the chances of people going somewhere without their phones are increasingly remote. The drawback to this approach is that if you say leave your phone on your desk while you walk to the water cooler, you will miss recording those steps. Simply slip the phone in your pocket, though, and you'll have a complete count.

For now, these sensors are only included as standard in high end expensive phone models. Both the Samsung S5 and the iPhone 5S include apps showing the steps their internal sensors report and there is a plethora of apps that build on the sensors to display more detailed analysis of your movement. And while the availability of these sensors is currently limited, if technology has taught us anything it is that prices fall rapidly - what was once the preserve of luxury models quickly permeates all price points. The addition of these sensors to more affordable models and even their inclusion in the big selling high end models means that the ability to track steps will be in more people's' grasp each day. Yet many people do not even realise that these features are built in to their phones and may either not take advantage of them, or purchase a dedicated activity tracker blissfully ignorant of their doubling up on sensors.

Activity monitors built in to phones offer several advantages:

- not another thing to buy
- not another thing to carry
- not another thing to charge
- once your phone is with you, it's with you
- it's not something you have to wear or remember to stick on
- it's not a fashion issue
- it's charged once you charge your phone
- doesn't require people to "carry or remember" another device

But they do have drawbacks too:

- while people these days are very reliant on their phones, they are often left nearby on desks or in handbags rather than being carried at all times - so some movement will be missed which may add up to be significant. For example, few people take their phone swimming, so something like a Misfit Speedo Edition or Withings Activitie that is fully waterproof will be a better choice for an avid swimmer looking to capture that work-out.
- Parents increasingly hand their phones to their kids to play with so the reported steps may reflect a hyperactive child's movement more than yours!
- it is dependent on your phone being charged to be active - with separate devices you can still track your steps even if your phone is dead and it will simply sync later

- tends to be high-end phones only that have motion sensors
- My phone just popped up a notification that I had been idle for over an hour and should consider moving. What it didn't know is that it had in fact been sat on the shelf of my treadmill while I covered 10K in the last 90 minutes. Now of course that doesn't matter as I've burned those calories whether the phone realized it or not, but it does show the dependency of internal phone sensors on the real situation to provide a holistic picture of activity.
- reliant on you having your phone on you at all times - if you leave it on the desk and move around, it's no use
- harder to use as a sleep monitor, although some do offer app-based solutions

It's worth spending a little time researching your activity tracker. You need one that delivers the features you want from a health point of view but also fits in your lifestyle - for example if you are more interested in swimming than running, you might want to prioritize waterproof models over anything else. And some of the wrist-worn ones are surprisingly uncomfortable for something that was supposedly designed to be on your wrist at all times other than when it's charging. You may also be surprised at the price range available. Fitness trackers can be had for as little as $20 right up to nearly $400. Studies show that the majority of fitness trackers are discarded by their users within six months. In fact, the Boston Globe recently reported on an initiative to collect and refurbish discarded trackers and redistribute them to under-privileged groups. This lack of longevity is not necessarily the fault of the tracker itself, but against the likelihood that their users will lose interest, it's important you choose the most suitable one to give yourself an improved chance of success so that there isn't any hardware-related excuse to quit.

As the technology matures and competition increases, the average price of activity trackers has been steadily decreasing. This has been dramatically illustrated by the arrival of the Xiaomi MiBand. This device compares favorably in terms of performance, accuracy and size with the more established market leaders and yet offers one of the longest batteries between charges.

When You Want More Information

Step tracking represents the simplest of motion sensor technology. Quite a lot of information can be gleaned from simple step data. The intensity of your activity will be clear as will the exact time you took your exercise and its duration, all recorded exactly by the app, either in real time or later when you pair your tracker and phone. The app can estimate the calories you burned as well as highlight the times you were idle. This is the extent of the information provided by the majority of trackers and it is huge in the detail it provides. If you download the raw data from your tracker it will show minute by minute recording of steps - every single one of them. But if you want to get a fuller picture of your activity, more advanced trackers include a number of other sensors to track even more attributes.

Step Into The Detail

If you ask most people what their cadence is, I reckon you'll be met with blank looks. Perhaps already very familiar to cyclists and hard core runners, it refers to the number of steps per minute. It is a good measure of your pace - the speed at which you are acquiring your steps and can reveal insights like the effect of terrain or tiredness on your activity. Along with cadence, more advanced trackers will monitor elevation and even the force with which your feet are hitting the ground.

As if we needed proof that sensors are available now quite literally from head to toe for every imaginable purpose, one company (Sensoria) is offering socks with sensors built in to them. Yes you read that right. Socks with sensors in them! The package includes an anklet that gathers impact data from the sock and transmits it to your phone. This enables extremely detailed measurement such as the amount of time your feet are in contact with the ground and the pressure/landing points of your feet. While it may seem like overkill in terms of data collection, it can help identify traits that may lead to injury or pain.

At time of writing the most advanced tracker I've tried is the Moov. This can be worn on either a wrist strap or an ankle strap. The claim is that by tracking the detail such as the G-Force with which your feet are hitting the ground, it can end the inaccurate and injury-inducing unsupervised workouts that derail the good intentions many people have when they set out on a fitness effort without having the necessary information to ensure it doesn't result in more harm than good. The second generation of Moov sees it reduce in price and physical size whilst switching from a rechargeable battery to a replaceable watch-type one that lasts for months.

Activity trackers come not only in all shapes and sizes (and colors too), but a new category of active devices is emerging. Rather than simply passively tracking your activity, the newer devices don't simply record the activity, they analyze it and offer real time advice on how you can improve. The virtual coach is an increasing level of sophistication being added to the more advanced tracking apps. Compared to the old days, pre-Smartphone, of simple pedometers, we can see a move from passive to active and from non-intrusive to instructional and even invasive. This takes the form of a voice in your ear as you walk/run that reports on your progress, the number of steps, your cadence, etc and provides motivation and encouragement in the form of hints and tips. My coach in Moov can vary from being helpful like "your cadence is slowing below target, try swinging your arms more vigorously" to the downright frightening "Your cadence is below target - imagine you are walking on hot coals"! Additional apps for this tracker target the tracking data and the coaching beyond running to swimming, boxing and cycling.

Beyond Steps

As activity trackers mature from their humble pedometer origins and expand their scope to feed more and more data to their accompanying smartphone apps you will see that what began as simple step counters now often include heart rate monitoring and more, many veering into full blown smartwatch territory to include notifications from your phone, as well as perhaps voice interactions with it.

While I still refer to the devices here as activity trackers, there are relatively few now that just track steps - the increasing sophistication makes it harder to classify them as merely activity trackers. Take for example Microsoft's plainly titled "Band 2". This device brings sensor overload to new heights but still costs less than $250 with the following plethora of sensors:

- Optical heart rate sensor
- 3-axis accelerometer
- Gyrometer
- GPS
- Ambient light sensor
- Skin temperature sensor
- UV sensor
- Capacitive sensor
- Galvanic skin response
- Barometer

Add to that you can track your sleep, pay for your coffee in Starbucks with the band, as well as check your email, messages and calendar and even access your virtual personal assistant if you're using one of Microsoft's phones. The Jawbone Up 4 also includes NFC technology so that you can pay for things with a flick of your wrist over the payment terminal in a shop - if I were to suggest a feature, I'd make sure you could only pay for health food!

The emergence of multi-purpose devices is likely to accelerate as a concept for several reasons, not least of which is for activity tracker manufacturers to defend against the inclusion of their core technology directly in phones. The fact that a band is in continuous contact with your skin gives them significantly more health-monitoring potential than a phone which may be in your pocket or bag for the majority of the day. Just as Microsoft chose to launch their first band with these advanced features, so too have Jawbone and Fitbit moved to add sensors that take advantage of their prime position on the body to deliver more insights and add to the debate about what attributes people will want to track.

If simply measuring steps isn't enough for you, there are multiple apps (with no additional hardware required) that can coach you through more involved workouts, with the added benefit of not tying you to a gym. Sworkit is a popular example boasting millions of downloads. It allows you to choose daily circuit training strength and cardio workouts, yoga, Pilates, and stretching with your choice of video routines from 5 to 60 minutes. The more adventurous can dynamically change the workouts to target specific body areas such as abs, back, butt, chest, hips, legs, stomach, thighs, etc with further personalization options to remove moves you can't do, or add rehabilitative ones in the case of injuries.

Analysis and Cross Reference

Regardless of the means you use to track the steps, a key component of the solution is the app that displays the steps and the associated software that adds value to the raw data, either in real time or at a later date. Activity trackers and their app can show you patterns and generate insights. They might be obvious when you think about it, but most people don't think about it. And they can be really good at pointing out how much exercise you actually do during the day, not only in a dedicated time but as part of your normal daily activity. My virtual "coach" pointed these patterns out to me. When presented with the data it's impossible to argue and it's kind of nice when the coach tells you you've done a good job! Increasingly, even as the trackers get more advanced and measure even more parameters, they are evolving to bring together information from more and more sources to create an increasingly comprehensive view of your well-being. So you'll see the same apps that appear here under Activity as companions to trackers appear again in the chapters on Diet, Sleep and Vital Signs and as we'll cover later, large companies like Apple and Google are looking to draw together information from multiple sources into a single repository.

Just collecting and presenting information isn't enough - there is a trick to how you present data: For instance, one of my apps reported that: "When you go to bed 30 minutes later than average, you tend to take 971 fewer steps the next day." I think there's something useful in that insight, but it's just not clear enough. But several days later, the app took another try and this time, it notified me: "Go to bed before 12:44 a.m. or you will likely get 10% less steps than an average day." Well, OK then!

Out of Favour

I mentioned earlier that many trackers are discarded by their users after a few months. This isn't just the finding of an abstract survey. Empirically, over the past couple of years, a number of my friends have experimented with activity trackers, much as many of them have flirted with various diet plans. And similarly to many diets, they have gone from enthusiastic adherence to waning interest to "falling off the wagon" completely. While some studies have shown that 30% of fitness trackers end up in drawers after 6 months, my own experience seems to indicate that it is frequently higher than that. Or maybe I just have very unmotivated friends!

Is this dropout rate a sign that the technology is not the great solution its proponents would have you believe? The truth is that this whole field is still young as a technology and is not yet able to deliver on all its promise. The best technology fades almost invisibly in usage and provides a real benefit to the user. This is true for most technology but may apply especially to more personal forms of technology such as wearable and health-related devices. Some point to the abandonment as an indicator that wearable tech is a passing over-hyped fad. More likely, it's no worse than the abandonment rate of diets and exacerbated by the first generation nature of many of these products.

I've investigated a little to see why people discard their activity trackers and have met a variety of answers, most of which are endemic to immature products:

- Simply lost interest
- Not fashionable
- Hard to use

- Don't consider the information it provides to be useful/actionable
- Disappointed it's not a magic cure
- Have to charge it too often
- Device is lost or damaged

Despite the inclination to give up on activity tracking, it's hard to think of a piece of technology that can inform, influence and assist more than mobile phones. Any technology that makes activity more fun, information, interesting, efficient, easy, affordable, or more effective is a good thing. But it takes willpower to turn it into a great thing.

Out of fashion?

Manufacturers are already adjusting their designs to address this kind of feedback. It hasn't taken long for trackers to be offered in all manner of colors to make them blend more with your outfit, as well as designer collaborations such as the Fitbit Tony Burch collection of decorative straps to make your FitBit into a style statement.

As a manufacturer of trackers, Misfit have perhaps put more effort into design than many others. Their flagship Shine product is already a very stylish and discreet minimalist aluminum disc and can be worn on a band or clipped on via a magnetic holder. They have also brought out a variant in conjunction with Swarovski that looks far more like jewelry than a utilitarian piece of technology with the reflecting crystals actually charging the device, removing the need for a replaceable battery. For those who prefer the less bling approach, they also produce a range of clothing such as T-Shirts and Socks with subtle little pouches to squirrel away your device as you go about your day.

One of the most advanced and expensive options aimed at the more serious athletes is the Hexoskin shirt. This $400 shirt has sensors embedded in it that relay a veritable dashboard of information including Cardiac (Heart Rate, HRV, Heart Rate Recovery, and ECG), Respiratory (Breathing Rate, Minute Ventilation (L/min) and Activity (Activity intensity, peak acceleration, steps, cadence and sleep positions) information.

Making Your Choice

With such an array of choices, some people may be dissuaded from making a choice simply as the risk of choosing incorrectly may be perceived to be too high. And while it's true that there is an increasingly large choice, it's also true that regardless of the form factor chosen, the awareness and associated focus it brings is what's important, much more so than the product itself. The lines between categories of products are blurring but that's nothing to be intimidated about - it means the chances of getting a product that suits your needs at a price you're willing to pay are increasing all the time.

Regardless of the form factor, remember that the associated apps are crucial. They will provide the visualization of your activity, the reminder if you're behind target and the ability to identify insights or to share the data with a professional. And the great thing with Apps is you can download them and have a look around before you commit to the hardware purchase, if you're not going to rely on the built in sensors in your phones. Do you like the app interface? Does it seem to offer the features you'd be interested in? There's no point in having great activity tracker hardware if you can't fathom the app or vice versa.

And for those who would like to try before they buy, US web service Lumoid (https://lumoid.com/wear) offers rental of 5 different models at a time to try, then you keep and purchase the one you want and simply return the others. If you think you may be interested in a gradual approach where you start with the basics and then may like the freedom to explore more details, be sure to pick an activity tracker that has features that can grow with you if you think you might get into exercise. Don't feel the need to over-spend at the start or buy something too complicated - keep in mind the likelihood is that a more advanced model with more features will be available at a lower price by the time you outgrow your current selection.

A word of warning when selecting your preferred tracker: despite them being engineered to be your constant companion and in many cases being water and shock proof, they do really show the punishment that the average human body goes through and remarkably emerges unscathed. A simple bang against something in a crowd might make you say ouch, sting for a moment or even bruise for a few days, but it can be fatal to a tracker!

Ultimately though, it doesn't matter how you count the steps; if technology of any kind helps keep you motivated to exercise more that's the most important thing. And remember that the steps counted are just numbers on your screen - if you rely on your phone to count steps and forget to bring your phone with you when you walk around to the shops, your body will count the steps even if it doesn't get reported back over Bluetooth or drawn in a graph or shared on Facebook.

Never Too Late!

There's some good news if you've been resisting activity and have perhaps convinced yourself it's not worth changing now - Regular exercise in old age has as powerful an effect on life expectancy as giving up smoking, researchers say. A study of 5,700 elderly men in Norway showed those doing three hours of exercise a week lived around five years longer than the sedentary. A French study showed similar cardiac benefits in men who started exercising at 40 as those who started at 30. However, while it is always recommended to consult a medical professional before undertaking any lifestyle changes, it is especially important in the case of older people who may want to embrace exercise.

Every Little Helps

If all this talk of exercise has made you tired, let me wrap up this chapter with one final thought on what constitutes activity and I promise not to mention "steps" again (for a while anyway). Non-Exercise Activity Thermogenesis (NEAT) is energy expenditure that you get from physical activities like cleaning, working, dancing, sleeping: in other words, unintentional exercise. These all count as activity and help burn calories. Bonus! But if you want to try to burn some more calories without even moving, there's some good news for you in a recent study….

Several studies have found that people who sit for the majority of their day live around two years less than those who are more active. Even if we deny it, most of us are guilty of huge quantities of sitting. We sit in the car or on the bus, at desks in work, and especially at home, where moving may only take the form of moving from one seat to another. Even as I write this paragraph, my watch has just alerted my wrist to the fact that I've been sitting for nearly an hour and it's time to stand up for a few minutes.

Standing up forces your body to use more energy than sitting down as your heart rate will be a little higher. Even if it is only about 10 beats per minute, that totals up to burn about 50 extra calories an hour. If you stand for even one hour a day for five days that's around 250 calories burnt a week which is 10,000 calories a year and not a step in sight! The impact of just 2,000 extra steps on health can be huge. A study published in 2007 in JAMA on the impact of pedometers showed that people who walk an average of 2,000 additional steps a day recorded a drop in their blood pressure of 3.8 mmHg over a period of 18 weeks. This reduces significantly the likeliness of a cardiovascular incident.

Hype or Panacea?

As with all emerging technologies, the consultants like to get in on the act predicting just how great an impact they foresee. The global revenues for smartphone-connected fitness tracking devices and equipment will grow from $2 billion in 2014 to $5.4 billion by 2019, according to a report from research firm Parks Associates. And Cisco estimate there will be half a billion wearable devices in use around the world within four years, including smart watches and fitness trackers - up from just 109m in 2014. Smart wearable devices may help save 1.3 million lives by 2020, according to a prediction made by Switzerland-based firm Soreon Research.

Personally, I'm not that interested in trying to predict how many devices there will be as I think it'll get harder to quantify them as the borders between current device categories blur away - I'm more interested in assessing how many people might be helped by any of the technologies that are becoming available.

If you just want to improve your overall activity level, then I'd absolutely not recommend you invest in sensor socks. But if you want to understand your running performance, potentially avoid injury and look for ways to improve your training efficiency, you'll probably stand to benefit more from a MOOV or Sensoria sock than a simple steps tracker as you likely well exceed 10k steps if you're a committed runner. If you're not sure about a tracker and have the discipline to record your key metrics yourself, then you can use an app to log your exercise manually and still have the benefits of sharing your achievements with friends, monitoring your trends and even gaining insights from top athletes. Apps such as Under Armour's Record can work with or without a tracker, as well as integrating with multiple data sources.

Staying in shape is a challenge and staying active is a key contributor. It goes against many trends of modern life - transport, convenience food and leisure that consists largely of watching either televisions on mobile devices, ironically the very mobile devices that could play a pivotal role in making our generation the healthiest ever.

So don't be put off by the 10,000 step target figure. It really is a lot of exercise if you think about it. But it's a target. And people miss targets all the time. What's important is that you're aware of it, tracking your progress towards it, and making lifestyle changes to help you get closer to the target. The 90 minutes of walking can be integrated into your day in small bursts of even ten minutes. The good thing about steps is that they are cumulative. Or you can increase the intensity of your activity if you're short on time. Multi-task too - Walk and Talk. Walk and listen. Steve Jobs used to go for walks with his senior executives rather than have sit down meetings.

And remember, you don't get fit or lose weight by tracking steps - you do it by taking them!

Chapter 5:
Food and Diet

In Chapter 3 Vital Signs, I mentioned that in some medical circles, weight or BMI is now often considered a vital sign. And indeed, it is undoubtedly one of the single biggest indicators and influencers of health. Unlike the other vital signs, it is not usually associated with urgent outcomes and hence does not have the dramatic appeal of paramedics shouting "BP 80 over 40" on TV. But over time, it has the ability to influence the other vital signs and in fact underlies or contributes to the emergence of a significant portion of potentially fatal conditions.

This book might be a bigger seller if I had called it "Your Phone Can Make You Thin". Such is the obsession with diets and weight-loss that every year, some $60 billion is spent on these targets in the US alone. At any given time, one in three people in the developed world is estimated to be on some form of a "diet". The good news is that your phone can in fact help to make you thin, but that's all it can offer - no miracle cure, no shortcut - just help. Apart from technology helping you, it's down to a combination of your exercise, eating habits and your microbiota (the trillions of microbes in your gut and how they interact with your body). So I'm afraid you can skip the rest of this chapter if you're looking for a miracle diet that somehow bypasses will power!

In the last chapter, we focused on activity and devices to help you quantify it. Yet while activity is an important part of a healthy lifestyle and a contributory factor to weight loss, ultimately it's disappointing how few calories non-intensive activity shifts - even the most generous of my activity tracking apps barely equates a 2 hour/15,000 step walk with a single McDonald's milkshake. But it's a fact so there's little point worrying about it - the main thing is to be aware of it and factor it into your dietary decision making. If you don't want to or can't embark on some rigorous exercise, shaking off calories after you eat is going to be hard. Then your only real non-surgical alternative is to tackle the other end of the issue - reduce your intake of calories. And that starts with awareness of exactly what, when and how you're eating.

Diets

A dreaded word for many that evokes images of starvation, drinking foul concoctions that taste as bad as they are good for you or following unpleasant eating regimes, diet is not a favored subject. Yet what we eat has an effect on our health and well-being second to almost none. But for all the New Year good intentions that millions embark upon each January, few of those diets will be adhered to, or be successful. History tells us that most people need help to achieve success through dieting. Before we explore the technologies aimed at understanding diet/weight loss, let's take a moment to describe the issues of what is overweight, is it really a problem and even if it is, is it my problem? Then we'll look at the wide range of technologies available, targeted at helping tackle this situation.

At this stage, it's also worth pointing out that while the largest health problem in many countries refers to overweight people, much of the technology we'll describe here is of use if you're underweight as it can equally help your awareness in tackling that problem.

What Constitutes Overweight?

Overweight and obesity are defined by an excess accumulation of fat in the body, usually due to an imbalance between caloric intake and energy expenditure. Or simply put, if you eat more than your body expends, you'll put on weight to the point of being overweight and eventually obese. Your body naturally uses up a certain amount of energy throughout the day, and you can use additional energy through exercise. You replenish your energy reserves through eating but if you eat more than you expend, the excess energy is stored in your body as fat. Remember though that the above is a general rule - everyone's body reacts differently to food and some extract more or less calories than average, and process/store nutrients in different ways.

As we will stress repeatedly in this book, everyone is individual and should look at their own particular circumstances before taking any action. In terms of general classifications of weight, what's the starting point? While most people are used to the concept of weighing themselves, absolute weight is not a useful measure without the context of your other physical attributes, such as height. Body mass index (BMI) takes account of an individual's height as well as weight and is widely used as a measure to define the line between desired weight level, overweight and obese.

The BMI is a body fat measurement defined as the ratio between a person's weight and the square of his or her height, generally expressed in kg/m^2. BMI is the most widely used measure for determining whether a given population suffers from overweight and obesity, as the same thresholds may be used for all adults, men or women. The WHO classification for BMI levels states that adults with a BMI equal or above 25 kg/m^2 are considered overweight and those over 30 kg/m^2 are considered obese. The scale applies to most people, though athletes or people with very high muscle concentration may erroneously seem overweight when assessed purely on BMI (due to its lack of focus on body fat percentage as opposed to muscle weight).

Is It Really A Problem?

The World Health Organization publishes a regular report called the "Global Burden of Disease", which measures the burden of disease around the world, comparing impacts of different diseases using the concept of disability-adjusted-life-year (DALY). This time-based measure combines years of life lost due to premature mortality and years of life lost due to time lived in states of less than full health. This is not necessarily a document that people outside of the healthcare and health policy-making circles are aware of and want to read, but it contains a number of interesting high level observations that should be of interest to us all and serve as an eye-opener if you've not really been aware of the scale of the challenges to our health.

According to the WHO, more than one billion adults worldwide are overweight or obese. Some estimates put the figure closer to 2 billion or as high as 1 in every 3 people worldwide. The WHO calculates that overweight and obesity are responsible for 44% of diabetes cases, 23% of instances of ischemic heart disease and 7 to 41% of certain cancers. Excess weight is therefore one of the five main mortality causes, along with high blood pressure, tobacco use, hyperglycemia (excessive blood glucose, usually associated with diabetes) and a lack of physical activity.

The CDC estimates that around $147 billion of annual medical costs are associated with obesity in the United States alone. And it's not just the US that faces this problem. "Poor diet is the leading modifiable risk factor for ill health in the UK". That is not the grandiose claim of a nutrition evangelist - it's the verdict from the WHO Global Burden of Disease Study.

If you want a less academic or global view of how humans are gaining weight, the fact that leading US manufacturer Humanetics recently had to increase the size of the crash test dummies to more accurately reflect the increasing average weight of humans does not reflect well on a society with the means at its disposal to be healthier than any previous generation. In fact it's an issue across too many countries to name separately here - the average diet in the western world contains too many calories, too much saturated fat, sugar and salt and too little fiber. And they are just the top-line nutritional categories. That's before you start to analyze if people are getting the recommended amounts of specific requirements...you know all those vitamins and minerals painstakingly listed on food labels but largely ignored!

UK NHS chief executive Simon Stevens has stressed the need to focus on preventing disease to ensure the very viability of the NHS in the future. And it's not just about money. If people ate more healthily, more than 33,000 premature deaths in the UK could be prevented each year. Being overweight is not just a question of vanity, body image or a lack of activity. It's not about being slim for the sake of it - it's important to state clearly I'm not advocating that everyone should be aiming for the stick-insect like physiques that have dominated much popular culture as somehow ideal. What I am highlighting is the need for people to strive for their healthy weight, not a mythical or media-contrived shape. The blunt health facts are that the number of major illnesses linked to being overweight should be enough to catch anyone's attention:

- Diabetes
- Heart disease
- High blood pressure
- Arthritis
- Indigestion
- Gallstones
- Some cancers (including breast and prostate)
- Snoring and sleep apnea
- Stress, anxiety, and depression
- Infertility

This list should be somewhat familiar as it shares many entries with the list in the previous chapter about the implications of a lack of exercise. Aside from the personal health issues, the worldwide financial cost of obesity is terrifying - it's about the same as smoking or armed conflict and greater than both alcoholism and climate change, research has suggested. The McKinsey Global Institute said it cost £1.3tn, or 2.8% of annual economic activity - it cost the UK £47bn.

"Well that's ok, but it's not my problem - I'm Not Fat, I'm big-boned!"

"Obese? Not me! So maybe I'm carrying a little more weight than is ideal but I feel fine and I'm not going to die from it." Most people are surprised when they are "suddenly" overweight. Typically, you gain weight quite gradually, virtually unnoticeably unless you are monitoring it. And if you're not aware of any problem you keep behaving as you were. We don't like to class ourselves as obese and while (eventually) acknowledging we're a few pounds heavier than we'd like to be, most do not see it as much more than an aesthetic bother and not something worthy of urgent action - diets always begin tomorrow! But whether we like it or not, weight is a very real issue.

While most people know that being overweight isn't a good idea, perhaps few are aware of (a) what exactly constitutes being over-weight and (b) the possible consequences of being overweight. People exhibit a remarkable capacity to convince themselves that they are not really or significantly overweight. They make excuses as to why, make plans to do something about it just as soon as X is out of the way or they fool themselves into thinking they aren't *really* over weight at all and sure they don't want to be like those skinny models anyway.

Is It Worth The Effort?

Make no mistake, technology assisted or not, sustainably losing weight is hard for most people. It requires changes to your behaviors, and lots of awareness and will-power. So is it worth all the hard work and is it going to genuinely help? The good news is that achieving the loss of just 5% of initial body weight produces clinically meaningful improvement in risk factors and for most people it can be achieved through lifestyle changes. Technology and specifically mobile technology can now supplement or take the place of costly third party interventions.

So What Can I Do?

Perhaps not surprisingly given the amount of consumer interest in this category and the large amounts of money spent in the quest for weight loss each year, this category has attracted significant attention from technology providers.

Just ahead of any enthusiastic urge you may have to dive into the numerous diet apps in the hopes of a quick fix, I would remind you that the most essential tool in this area is the weighing scales. This is the only way to establish your baseline and monitor progress driven by the various interventions you may choose and which may in turn be assisted by technology.

The Connected Scales

As we saw a little earlier in Chapter Three Vital Signs, the once humble bathroom scales has been supplanted by a more advanced affair that now features Bluetooth, WiFi, atmospheric sensors and even the ability to tell you the weather! The most advanced models record not only your weight, but your BMI and Body Fat % (and several other parameters in some models), displaying the results on a large screen where the needle used to be. The key thing is that they transfer this information to the companion app on your phone wirelessly, as well as to a secure storage area in the cloud.

Having this information accurately recorded and visualized shows you any trends clearly and plays a crucial role in narrowing down the causality of any changes, be they good or bad, when combined with additional information sources. Scales are a great starting point for adding some technology to your routine - as using them needs no expertise! In fact, your current weight is the first thing that most health-related apps ask you when you set up a new account on them. When considered along with your age, gender and average activity level, it's the starting point to determine your recommended daily calorie intake. This figure will vary based on whether you are trying to gain, lose or maintain weight.

Choosing a scale is not quite as complicated as choosing an activity tracker. Thankfully, there is only a handful of models and core feature sets are very similar. You can choose to spend a little extra to gain more measurement capabilities that may appeal to people looking for deeper insights to guide their dietary interventions.

Once you've established your baseline weight and desired target weight, most apps will recommend a daily calorie intake and an exercise regime. We'll talk a lot more about exercise in the activity chapter, but for now, let's focus on calories.

Calories

Calories as a word is part of everyday language. I think it's fair to say that most people know in general that eating too many of them is bad, things that taste nice tend to have lots of them and exercising uses them up faster than doing nothing. But while researching this book and painstakingly recording the calories I was consuming, I began to wonder a little more about calories - what are they and what is the actual relationship between calories and weight?

A calorie is actually a measure of energy, just as a volt is a measure of electricity, a kilogram is a measure of weight and a litre is a measure of liquid volume. Technically a calorie indicates how much energy it takes to change the temperature of 1 gram of water by 1 degree Celsius.

The human body needs energy to do anything but it is also remarkably energy efficient. It runs on surprisingly little "fuel" each day. Just how much it needs depends on many factors including what you do during a day (sleep all day, exercising, whatever). The average adult male needs between 2,000 and 2,500 calories a day. So if he eats this amount of energy a day he should neither gain nor lose weight as he would be consuming as much he uses. Of course the amount of calories needed per day varies from person to person and day to day, as does the amount of calories that each of our bodies can extract from the same food, so remember that all references to calories are only a guide and cannot be applied equally to everybody.

So where do these calories go? The amount of calories your body needs is the total amount of energy required for its normal operations - your heart to pump, your lungs to fill with air, your body to keep warm, your hair to grow, your stomach to digest food and all those things you generally don't think about in a day. This is known as the basal metabolic rate. This is what your body would need regardless of what activities you do. Generally speaking the larger you are, the higher your basal metabolic rate. Think about it: a 100 pound woman needs less energy to breath and pump her heart than a 300 pound man. This is no different than thinking of the amount of fuel a Ford Focus needs to cover the same distance relative to say a BMW X5.

If we take an average male whose body consumes around 2000 calories per day and he eats 2200 calories on a given day, he has consumed 200 calories more than required to keep his body operating. The problem is that these 200 calories are still in the body. And since they are not used up quickly, they will be stored somewhere: that somewhere is fat. A pound of fat stores 3500 calories or 1 kilogram stores 7700 calories. So to put a calorie number on weight loss, to lose a pound (.45kg) of fat *in a week*, a person needs to eat approximately 500 fewer calories per day than they expend.

How Many Calories Are In That?

Calories are invisible and not necessarily directly related to the size of the food in question. How good are people at estimating calories? Not very, according to a Harvard Medical School study of more than 3,400 customers at fast food chains published in the British Medical Journal in 2014. The study concluded that people significantly underestimated the calories in their meals with more than 25% of people underestimating calorie content by at least 500 calories.

Perhaps you reckon you're better than average at estimating calories? Let's do an exercise - look at your last supermarket shopping list, estimate the number of calories in each item and then check the label on each item to see what the true numbers are. Research shows you are likely to vastly underestimate the contents of each item. Doctors warn a large glass of wine can contain around 200 calories - the same as a doughnut. Yet the Royal Society for Public Health says the vast majority of people are blissfully unaware. Packaged food comes with calorie information, but alcohol is exempt from EU food labelling laws and when you're in a restaurant it's rare to see calorie content or portion weight displayed on a menu.

If you are going to rely on the calorie counts you're reading on food labels, how do you know that they are accurate? If you've ever wondered how food companies come up with calories for the nutrition facts panel? The system they use is called the Atwater Method. Food is burned in a device called a "calorimeter." and the amount of heat energy released is used to heat water. Remember, 1 calorie is the amount of energy required to heat one gram of water by 1 degree.

While this gives a good indication, it doesn't work uniformly across all food types, and in fact humans don't fully extract all calories from all types of food as we digest them. Cooking and food processing methods also affect how readily our bodies can extract calories from food. Nor do all humans extract calories from food with the same efficiency - our individual microbiome (naturally occurring bacteria in our gut) has a big impact on this. And given that natural ingredients will always vary, it's good to remember that labelled calorie counts are legally compliant if they are +/- 20% of the actual value. And while that may not seem a like a large variation, over time a seemingly small variation adds up to fairly meaningful amounts - a variation of just 50 calories per day in how much we eat, or in how efficient our extraction of calories from food is, equates to 2kg per year or 20kg in ten years.

Menu Display - Nanny State or Informed Choice?

New legislation in Ireland requiring restaurants to display the calorie content in the same size font as price on menus was met with applause from the Royal College of General Practitioners but greeted with howls of protest from the Restaurant Association of Ireland who claimed it would have a devastating impact on their members. Bemoaning it as a nanny state tactic, the scheme's detractors seem to miss the point that people are still free to eat as many calories as they wish - all the measure does is to give people the information that may help them to make healthier choices. I fully expect most people will carry on regardless - but shouldn't restaurants seek to be transparent with their customers rather than relying on ignorance? In any event, as customers increasingly have mobile tools at their disposal, they will be able to assess a menu themselves and estimate its contents.

Just as the smoking ban was heralded as the death-knell for the hospitality sector, people have adapted and those who want to smoke are free to do so outside. Those who want to eat in restaurants but make informed choices about what they are eating should also be empowered to do so. There must also be a consideration of the greater good. Restaurants cannot expect to continue to serve demonstrably unhealthy portion sizes with impunity. Pressure will likely increase in the coming years beyond what technology can do - for example, political influence already extends to banning unhealthy food promotion near schools. The implications of who knows what you are eating, beyond you and your healthcare professional will be discussed in a later chapter.

Tracking Your Caloric Intake

Monitoring your calorie intake and regulating it based on reaching a target number isn't new - calorie controlled diets have been around since 1918. Food diaries have long been the staple of such calorie controlled weight loss programs, as have weekly meetups with support groups for group discussion of progress. But as technology evolves, the smartphone is emerging as the centerpiece of these counting activities.

There are a number of technologies we'll consider here:

- App to track calories/Apps with barcode scanners
- Scanner to assess food content
- Wristband to sense inputs

There's no shortage of apps that track what you eat. Most simply enable you to record what you had for each meal, as well as any snacks in between. The better apps have extensive databases of food and their associated calories (as well as detailed information on micronutrients) while bar code scanners are included to make it quicker to identify packaged foods without the need to search for specific products.

If you eat a lot of packaged food, it is genuinely quick to scan or search for items and add them to your meal list. This gives you a daily total of the calories consumed, based on the values in the app's database. If you tend to eat less prepared food and work more with your own ingredients, tracking your calories is more challenging. You can estimate the amount of each ingredient and search for it in the database or use an enhanced kitchen scale such as the PrepPad which combines weight with an app that calculates nutritional content.

Food tracking apps typically remind you during the day to enter your meals data, with helpful tips popping up if you don't input straight after mealtimes such as "it's easier to record as you go along". And while these reminders are useful during the day, they only apply to set mealtimes. If you're a snacker, you need to be honest and input the snacks you eat each day. You can of course cheat calorie tracking apps so that you like the total number at the end of each day, but you can't cheat your body!

Lifesum and MyFitness Pal are two of the most popular food tracking apps. Both offer streamlined interfaces to input your meals, split into Breakfast, Lunch, Dinner and Snacks as main categories. Comprehensive food databases can be searched, or you can input by scanning barcodes on packaged foods. Links to activity tracking apps give you credit for any exercise or you can enter exercise sessions manually if you don't have an activity tracker, and both apps offer trends and insights on your consumption patterns.

Is calorie tracking an effort? Yes there's no denying that it is, initially at least. But routine helps and I have to say I now automatically reach for my phone after a meal to quickly input the details. But more than that, I've found being aware of calories makes me think twice before choosing my food so that I make the most of the calories I'm targeting each day. And the most important question - is it worth the effort? Are those 2 or three minutes spent inputting your food, finding healthier substitutes or gaining actionable insights not worth improved health?

People I've asked whether they'd consider tracking calories protest that it's time consuming. Recording what you eat can definitely be tedious. After each meal you have to remember to input and record what you had. Different apps have different databases but it takes less than two minutes per meal in reality. Most apps maintain a list of frequent foods so it gets quicker to record as you repeat previous meals (which most people tend to).

Yet what could be more important than investing in your health. Can any of us truly say we don't have 2 minutes extra to record the contents of a meal? If anybody was asked to find two minutes more to eat, I have little doubt that they would. They would wait two minutes more to be served or two minutes more to get the bill. At the end of the day, what gets measured gets managed as most leading business consultants will tell you. And I would argue that while you should track what you eat, it's not important down to every last calorie. For anyone who gives up just because it's too hard to track everything down to the last calorie, I would say just track to the nearest hundred calories rather than give up - approximation is better than ignorance. The benefits are the awareness, the vigilance, the second thoughts, the conscious, informed decision making. As I started tracking my calories, I found myself checking the calorie cost of a treat before I went to eat it and I quickly started to reappraise treats relative to each other - some I considered more "worth it" than others. When you can assess the relative calorie cost of each item, you can make better decisions on the taste/benefit to additional effort required analysis!

So what if you decide to supersize things in McDonalds. It's very tasty, so why not - but at least know it requires a two hour walk to make a dent and burn off some of those delicious calories. I would also contend that it gets easier. Scan barcodes, repeat frequent meals, search a vast database of products. Or manual entry based on what's printed on the package is something you get very used to as you come to rely on your app more and more.

Is it easier to record and manage your food than finding time for exercise? While it's not an either/or situation (you should really have a healthy diet and get exercise), making changes to your food consumption doesn't require any exertion. Just an awareness of what foods to eat, in what quantities and perhaps an additional element of planning/care in selecting and purchasing. Changing your diet for the better involves a relative few actions - reducing portions, minimizing snacks or replacing them with healthier alternatives.

I wish I had more good news for people who are struggling towards a healthier weight, but I don't. Losing weight is hard. Keeping it lost is hard too. All help is welcome, and undoubtedly technology will help some people. And whether it's tracking food or planning what you want to eat, there is a plethora of apps to make you think more about how the day is portioned out (pun intended) - breakfast - importance of good start, main meal at lunchtime and less in the evening.

But this is an area where while you can control your own inputs some of the time, it's not easy when you're out. So you may need to support political change. Ireland's recent move to legally require calories on menus is a good start. If restaurants and takeaways defaulted to smaller portions, it would help as people habitually keep eating until their plates are empty, even if they are already full.

Tracking without the Effort - There's an Appcessory for that

If you are interested in tracking calories but can't be bothered with the hassle of inputting what you eat into even the most streamlined of calorie tracking apps, you may be heartened to hear of one gadget that was demonstrated at the Consumer Electronics Show in Las Vegas in January 2015, and subsequently made available for sale in mid-2015. The Healbe GoBe is a wrist-worn device that claims to track your body's calorie intake and expenditure without you having to tell it what you're eating.

This is a first generation product and in its current form is quite bulky and priced at the higher end of the wearable technology market at $299. But it is undoubtedly intriguing and a glimpse of the range of sensors that will continue to be squeezed into a single device. Not only does it track calories, it also tracks steps, distance travelled, sleep, stress, heart rate and even blood pressure. It remains to be seen how ultimately accurate it is but in my tests, it seems to estimate calories reasonably well, within 15-20% of my own estimates. That is sufficient to help you understand your eating behaviors and provides enough relative accuracy to spot trends and impacts. The attraction of not having to pause to input foods or guess the contents means it may appeal to a different segment of user who wishes to become more health conscious. Whatever the debate about the accuracy, it has an uncanny knack of knowing that I've eaten something - frequently prompting me with "were you eating between x and y o'clock" - only for me to realize that I did indeed eat at that time but that I may have forgotten to log the food in my normal tracking app. Even that reminder from the Healbe app increases awareness and visibility of my eating patterns which I might otherwise forget. As an all-in-one well-being device, it is the current leader in the number of parameters tracked for the least user effort.

How Does it Work?

This new application of mobile technology fits firmly in the category of seeming to be too good to be true - a wristband that tracks what you're eating without you having to do anything? Could this really be the solution to removing one of the biggest barriers that stops people recording their diet?

The HealBe uses a proprietary technology to estimate what's going on in your body as you digest food. It is based on how your body processes what you eat. 10-15 minutes after you eat, your body starts converting the carbohydrates in your food into glucose. This process continues for up to 4-6 hours, depending on what you eat and your body's unique physiology. As glucose concentrations rise, your cells absorb glucose and release water. Fat and protein in your food influences the rate of glucose absorption—leading to different shapes and durations of the "glucose curve," which the device measures using an impedance sensor that tracks the fluid moving in and out of your cells. A clever algorithm then analyzes these impedance readings and calculates calorie intake based on your glucose curves.

As well as its main focus on automated calorie tracking, the multi-purpose HealBe GoBe measures movement the same as many of the activity trackers that we talked about in the earlier chapter. It also manages to track blood pressure and heart rate.

Finding Alternative Foods

Apart from learning that you probably aren't very good at estimating calories if you've not previously shown any interest in them, you may also be surprised that many of the foods you like contain high calories or other undesirable ingredients. But before you give up, consider that you may simply need to substitute a similar product for the one you've traditionally chosen. Most of us are creatures of habit when it comes to buying produce and rarely switch. But sometimes similar products have quite different ingredients or portion sizes.

If you need help substituting healthier foods - you probably won't be surprised to know that there is an app for that….it helps you identify healthier near substitutes for the food you're buying. And there can be surprising differences in apparently similar products. Scan the barcode on a product and the app will offer you alternatives - for each product, it will display substitute products and the details in terms of how much less calories each option contains. So with a simple barcode scan, you can replan your weekly shopping and come away with a similar shopping basket but with a reduced calorie total.

Foodswitch UK is a free app that offers two modes of operation - FoodSwitch and SaltSwitch. In FoodSwitch mode it will show you lower calorie or healthier options when you scan a product. In the SaltSwitch mode, it is designed to focus more on suggesting alternatives with lower salt content for people who are trying to manage high blood pressure.

Fooducate is a detailed food resource that provides nutritional information and suggestions of healthier alternatives when you scan a barcode and grades food on a scale of A- D, based on the advertised nutritional content and level of processing. It also features personalized information to track allergies and highlights information that may be on packaging but not obvious such as excessive sugar, trans fats, MSG and food colorings.

Drinking

I'd say if I asked most of my friends how their phone could save their lives when it comes to drinking, they would clamor to tell me about the latest app they have that details how to make great cocktails or point to an app that matches wine perfectly to any ingredient you care to name. And while it's true that there are many such apps available, that's not really what I have in mind for this section….

The Importance of Water

Just as most people know that they should eat healthily, it's widely known that it is advised to drink lots of water each day. Just as with steps, people may be surprised to know that the current best medical advice is that everyone should drink 2 liters of water per day. That's a fairly sizable requirement, and typically requires a level of awareness and planning before it can become a routine standard part of your day.

Depending on which study you believe, the human body is made up of between 45% and 65% water. Large individual variations are driven by age, sex, and adiposity (fat) but even if you take the lowest estimated figure, water is still the largest single compound in the body. It would be foolish to underestimate the importance of water for the correct functioning of our bodies. When you drink enough, it makes you feel full, distributes nutrition around your body and removes toxins. Dehydration, or the loss of water, can have serious consequences if you do not replenish the water you lose through breathing, sweat and excretion. Losing five to eight percent of your water level can cause fatigue and dizziness. Over ten percent can cause physical and mental deterioration, accompanied by severe thirst. A decrease more than fifteen to twenty-five percent of the body's water is usually fatal.

Water can help with weight loss by reducing feelings of hunger - you feel fuller for an hour longer if you have water with dinner. A bit like the daunting steps target of 10,000 per day, the recommended daily amount of water intake is also steep! Several of the apps I've tried have suggested I need to drink upwards of 2 liters per day. Although it seems a lot, if you keep a water bottle as a companion and opt to drink water before and with meals, you can get through it. Focusing on water consumption has forced me to cut down on my caffeine, which comes with a double benefit as caffeine in large doses is usually considered a diuretic - a substance that increases water loss.

Available alongside as separate apps or integrated with food tracking apps, there is a number of digital ways to track your water consumption. Hydration is an important parameter in itself, but it can also play a significant role in diet. If you drink enough water before a meal, it can moderate how much food you eat. If you're already using a food tracking app, it's probably easiest to use any water tracking facilities it has. If you're not yet using a food tracking app or are only interested in your water consumption, you can choose a dedicated water tracking app. I have tried a quantity tracking water bottle that displays the amount of water you've consumed on a little screen on the front of the water bottle but I found the lack of integration and reporting to my phone to render it ineffective. Then along came the HidrateMe, a connected water bottle and app that tracks your water intake and glows to make sure that you never forget to drink your water again. And if you need to keep track of more liquids than water, entrepreneurs have created the first smart drinking cup - the Vessyl can identify whatever liquid you put in it and record the liquid calories via its app.

Which Diet is for me?

Although dieting is often treated as a simple question of eating less, it is vital to consult a health professional before making any radical dietary changes. The authors of a 2007 JAMA review warned that "[i]t is possible that even moderate calorie restriction may be harmful in specific patient populations, such as lean persons who have minimal amounts of body fat". As with all other areas of discussion in this book, weight is not a simple topic with a single solution. If you struggle with weight issues (under as well as over), then seek professional help.

I'm not going to discuss the relative merits of different types of diet plans - Wikipedia quotes that a meta-analysis (which is a statistical method for contrasting and combining results from different studies) of six randomized controlled trials found no difference between the main diet types (low calorie, low carbohydrate, and low fat). It's your choice to find what works for you. But there is likely a smartphone-based app to help you stick to any diet and more importantly to help you understand the impact that diet is having on your physical condition. My view of dieting is that it's not all about sacrifice - it's more about priorities. If you do want to indulge, then you need to exercise to earn back the credits.

Non Digital Tricks

While this book is about the potential impact of mobile technologies on well-being, it would be myopic to ignore the importance of non-digital behaviors to successful outcomes. But while not wanting to stray from the core premise, these non-digital tips are among the kinds of advice that diet-related apps are likely to give you that may help you see the numbers you want appear on your screen!

- Eat bread one slice at a time rather than as a closed sandwich - this makes the meal take longer and seem like more
- Get smaller plates - a proven psychological trick - this fools the brain into thinking it's had enough
- Only have two courses for dinner instead of three - skipping starter or dessert probably won't leave you hungry but makes it much easier to stay the right side of the calorie curve
- Empty a portion of sweets or crisps into a bowl - don't always feel you have to finish the packet
- Watch out for portions -as they are on the increase - the average bagel 20 years ago was 140 calories. Today's average bagel is a whopping 350 calories or more than 2.5 times the size it used to be.

It's Also How You Eat

With all the emphasis and support available to monitor your intake, you might think that is job done. Unfortunately, it's not just what you eat, but how you eat too that can have a big impact on your well-being. The right food eaten in the wrong way can offset some of the potential benefits of maintaining a good diet.

It's Not All About The Calories

If you're a bit tired of talking about calories, I understand! Let's move on....while the caloric and nutritional content of the foods you eat are vital considerations, they aren't the only ones. Other factors impact the effect that these inputs have on your body. For example, the time and speed at which you eat is also important. Help is at hand here too from technology, if these are areas you want to address.

Research has shown that the speed at which you eat impacts. Yet again, there is technology available to help manage this and focus attention on it. Although not perhaps as big a focus as other areas of nutrition, for those truly dedicated to making the most of it, this additional step may be useful. Monitoring the speed of your meals has a couple of positives. Better digestion, less likelihood to over-eat.

So far, I've come across two technologies designed specifically to work with your mobile phone to give you more information on how you eat, and impact your approach to eating.

- Although people I know are well used to me having strange gadgets, one of the most unusual ones has to be my HAPI Smart Fork. Yes, a fork that you need to charge! A fork that uses Bluetooth to connect to your phone and report on your eating, a fork that even vibrates if you eat at a faster rate than best practice recommends. I can't pretend that having your fork vibrate isn't an unusual sensation! But it definitely draws your attention to the speed at which you tend to shovel food into your mouth. The app displays detailed timing metrics such as how many servings you've taken, what the interval between mouthfuls is compared to what it should be and how many times you've managed to take the right gap between servings. Somewhat ironically, I just had another app advise me against using my phone or playing games while I eat as apparently people are more likely to eat too much when distracted by technology. Its advice? Eat with people as the conversation will likely make you eat more slowly. I guess that app didn't know I had a fork for that ;)

- Another device called the BitBite takes a different approach but is also focused on the how element of eating. This crowd-funded gadget comes in the form of a small ear-piece. It is designed to encourage you to slow down, chew more and eat at regular intervals. It monitors eating patterns by analyzing chewing sounds so it knows when, where, what and how the user is eating. Analysis of this data then sends you real-time dietary advice on how to eat healthier.

Food Quality

It's not only the quantity of the food you consume or the pace at which you consume it that matters - the quality matters too. It is hard to know the exact extent of food-related illnesses as many people do not report mild instances, and in other cases, the incubation period of the illness may make definitive association with a cause difficult. In the US, there are over 200,000 cases of foodborne illness every day. While the best defense against such outbreaks is good personal and food handling hygiene as well as thorough cooking, there is now a device that can analyze your ingredients and warn you if it has started to spoil and therefore likely to cause an illness.

When it comes to assessing the quality of your food, there are two mobile technologies that can help - one to look at the composition of your food, and one to test the freshness:

- Recently funded via a crowdfunding campaign, the Tell Spec device is a handheld scanner that can report on the composition of food that you point it at. That's right, point this device at an item of food, and the app will tell you the fat, protein, sugar and gluten content. It is a miniaturized spectrometer - a device that uses reflected light waves to determine what it's looking at based on different wavelengths. So even if you aren't sure what a food is, this device will let you decide if it matches your dietary requirements.

- The descriptively named Food Sniffer is a small handheld scanner that can detect if certain food types have started to spoil. Over 100 volatile organic compounds (VOCs) are emitted by decomposing beef, poultry, and fish; simply pointing the Food Sniffer device at these food types enables you to see on the App if the spoiling process has begun. It will advise you to cook the meat extra thoroughly if the process has only just begun or advise you not to consume it at all if it detects levels that are too high.

The next time you see someone in a restaurant pointing their phone at their plate, they may not be one of those people who put incessant food images on Instagram - in the near future, perhaps someone pointing their phone at their plate will be assessing the quality of their food, its ingredients, its caloric content, its suitability for their preferred diet/allergenic profile and not just adding a photo of it to the social network of their choice to brag to their friends.

Personalized Nutrition Coaching

Of course not everyone will find that tracking their food intake is an effective means of improving their diet. In some cases, people may respond better to personalized information, the opportunity to ask questions involving their own food preferences and experiences, and even regular oversight from a trusted professional. We would probably all secretly like to have a personal trainer and nutritionist. It sounds glamorous, but also effective. Someone who is dedicated to improving us and who will adapt to our specific needs. They will provide the guidance, motivation and encouragement. It's a handy excuse as few can afford a personal trainer but can convince themselves easily that without a bespoke plan, they are doomed to fail and therefore better not to try. But now your very own personal trainer and nutritionist is only an app away. The final group of apps I want to cover in this section comprises services that turn your mobile into your very own eating coach.

- The HAPICoach app (from the makers of the Hapi SmartFork) brings you 1:1 nutrition coaching where you send pictures of your meals to the coach and get feedback. The app also shares any other information you choose from other devices such as blood pressure monitor, activity trackers and scales.

- Services like Rise offer you a real life qualified nutritionist who will assess your meals and give you feedback, at a cost of about $2 per day. Alternatives such as Lark, use a computer to analyse your data (you can share your Apple Health data for example) and give you advice. It's personalized based on your data but fairly formulaic in terms of the responses and advice it can give. Still it does simulate an external party reviewing your data and holding you to account.

These days, you can get a subscription box for just about anything and now that includes customized nutritional supplements. The data available from your activity trackers can also be combined with additional information sources such as either your DNA information (if available) or a lifestyle questionnaire to create a personalized nutritional plan. Providers in this customized nutritional space include Nutrimatix which offers customized science-based, vitamin and supplement advice based on data gathered via your fitness tracker and questionnaire information. Using the app, you can share the recommendations with your medical professional doctors, generate shopping lists or order custom-blended powdered drink formulas directly from Nutrimatix. Wellpath offers a similarly customized service, but adds the ability to link to your profile from genetic service 23andme, as well as automated amendments to your monthly supplement deliveries (available in pill and/or powder formats) as your data inputs change.

The Benefits of Information

The ease of tracking your weight and your food on your smartphone should give you the real-time information you need to make the right decisions. If your weight is going up, check the foods you've been eating and adjust accordingly by eating less or exercising more. The instant visibility should help you stay motivated as you can identify and replicate good days, and modify the behaviors on bad days. It is surprising how little consideration most people give to what they put into their bodies. People have a great ability to kid themselves that they are sticking to a diet. However, once you record your meals (and yes, that bar of chocolate counts!!), it's hard to argue with the stark facts.

At the risk of oversimplification, I like the way nutrition information is presented in the Jawbone Up app that accompanies their activity tracker. This app categorizes food into three basic groups:

- All you can eat
- Don't over do it
- Pass on these

Although it is probably not the categories of food they teach at nutrition school there's a lot to be said for categories that people can understand and that can bring actionable insights to the public at large. This light-touch level of advice may seem less oppressive than some of the more rigorous apps and serves to highlight the variety of approaches available.

In the case of good/bad food choices though, it's not always attributable to a lack of knowledge. Most people do know that fruit and vegetables are good for you, and confectionery or candies are not. But the majority of people are surprisingly poor at putting our knowledge of a healthy diet into practice. Driven by a lack of interest, time pressures, habit and a general belief it can be dealt with later many continue to make very bad food choices on a daily basis. Although we like to think of ourselves as rational, intelligent people who make good decisions, research shows much of our behavior in relation to food or indeed physical activity, is not a conscious, deliberative act. Rather, it is an automatic response, shaped by the circumstances in which we find ourselves and the environment and social cues that surround us.

Culturally it can be unacceptable not to eat what you're given, and restaurants are generally guilty of a one size fits all (except children's menu) policy on portions and routinely ask "what's wrong" if you fail to finish your meal. I've not yet seen anyone reply with "you gave me twice the recommended daily amount of calories in that one course of one portion of one meal of the day" but it might well be true.

But for people who are surprised they are not losing weight, or indeed are gaining it, the objective facts presented by an App are a strong counterpoint to the more attractive perspective offered by friends "sure you have to eat" and the like. Combining technologies can be the most powerful solution. Pairing the discipline of recording calories with the quantifiable numbers on your connected scales removes the ability to argue away anomalies and is most likely to support your weight management efforts with the right motivational levels of actionable information.

Chapter 6:
Sleep

"Sufficient sleep is not a luxury—it's a necessity—and should be thought of as a 'vital sign' of good health."

- CDC, Centers for Disease Control and Prevention

If what we eat and how much we exercise are very much individual daily choices, one thing we all have in common is the need for sleep. In fact, we spend around a whopping one third of our entire lives asleep. It is vital to our well-being, both physical and mental; providing time for our body to recharge, process and prepare. Yet few of us put much effort into ensuring the quality of our sleep or make a significant effort to ensure we get enough. In fact, we are more likely to complain about being tired but remain unwilling to forgo the last bit of TV watching late at night; leaving too few hours between going to bed, actually falling asleep and the dreaded alarm the next morning….

Although most of us take what sleep we do get for granted, a very large number of people struggle to sleep each night (estimated by National Institute of Neurological Disorders and Stroke, at about 40 million people in the United States suffering from chronic long-term sleep disorders each year and an additional 20 million people experiencing occasional sleep problems). An even greater number don't get the recommended amount of sleep. In a recent Royal Philips survey of nearly 8,000 people in 10 countries, 96% said that good sleep is valuable to them, and 57% admitted their sleep could be better but they hadn't taken action to improve sleep. In the US, the first-ever federal health study about sleeping pill usage recently found that nearly nine million Americans take prescription sleeping pills, despite the associated health risks of trying to chemically enhance sleep.

There is a very wide variety of reasons for people not getting enough sleep and while the human body is remarkably resilient in terms of operating on sub-optimal levels of sleep, there are undoubted health implications associated with poor sleep, as well as the more obvious day to day performance challenges it brings. To date though, sleep has received significantly less attention as a source of poor health or a contributor to good health than diet and exercise.

Before we go through the technologies now widely available to help us better understand sleep, let's take a quick look at sleep in a bit more detail so we understand what we are trying to track, as well as the known or purported implications of not getting enough sleep.

The Importance of Sleep

Despite a common need for regular sleep, we are all different when it comes to how much and when we sleep. Most people need 7½ to 8 hours of sleep. But some people are "short sleepers" who only need 6 hours of sleep a night or less. On the other hand, some people are "long sleepers" who need at least 9 hours of sleep a night. When I say "need", what do I mean?

So how much sleep do we need? A simple and cogent but perhaps seemingly flippant answer is - enough to feel refreshed and energetic. However, scientific/medical understandings of why we sleep are still imperfect. Some of the influences that underlie sleep are well established. How long someone has been awake is clearly relevant, with performance declining, and sleepiness developing for most people after about 16 hours of being awake. The time of day also affects the tendency to sleep, if sleep is needed. Such pressure to sleep is greatest at 4 to 6 am and 2 to 4 pm, at which points in time traffic accidents that are sleep-related peak. Age influences sleep need as well. Sleep requirements remain unaltered but, with age, there is less ability to stay asleep and there is an increased tendency to nap in the day.

The advent of the Electroencephalogram (EEG) has enabled scientists and researchers to measure brain activity during sleep and has given us an understanding that sleep is not just one continuous status of not being awake. Scientists have observed two distinct types of sleep, rapid eye movement (REM) and non rapid eye movement (NREM) enter the sleep cycle after 90 to 100 minutes. The transition into sleep is through an orderly progression from light to deep non REM sleep to REM dreaming sleep, repeated a number of times throughout the sleep period in question, usually one night. In REM sleep, during which dreaming is common, the body is literally and physically paralyzed to prevent acting out of dreams, unless of course you're a sleepwalker.

Not All Sleep Is Equal

Most apps that track sleep provide nice graphs showing the different phases. Interpreting these can be a little tricky so it's useful to understand a bit more about sleep cycles. If you're keen to know more, then check out the details at the American Academy of Sleep Medicine (AASM.org) website.

As I said before, I don't want to medicalize or over-scienceify things, but the more you look into seemingly simple things like sleep, you being to realize just how complicated it really is, and just how little we actually know about it. So rather than spend too long examining sleep, I'll cover off the concepts you need to know to begin to understand it a bit more.

In normal parlance, sleep is a fairly general term that encompasses several cycles over the hours that you're asleep. Human sleep occurs in periods of approximately 90 minutes, which include an increasing proportion of REM sleep as they repeat. This rhythm is called the *ultradian sleep cycle*. Sleep proceeds in cycles of REM and NREM, usually four or five of them per night depending on how much time you spend trying to sleep. The AASM divides NREM into three stages: N1, N2, and N3, the last of which is also called delta sleep or slow-wave sleep. The whole period normally proceeds in the order: N1 → N2 → N3 → N2 → REM. Body temperature, heart rate, breathing rate, and energy use all decrease with deeper sleep.

Stages N1 and N2: 50% of total sleep, i.e. 4 hours per night. Stage N1 corresponds to the falling asleep phase during which we are neither completely asleep nor completely awake. Body movements are sporadic. Stage 2 corresponds to a light sleep phase during which we have dreams that make us feel as though we are awake. In this phase of sleep, we can be awoken by light noises.

Stages N3 and N4 represent approximately 25% of total sleep, i.e. 2 hours per night. They correspond to a very deep sleep, where the person is completely still. There is very little brain activity or reaction to external stimuli. Heart rate and breathing are slow and regular, and the face is expressionless. Deep sleep phases are crucial times for the body to regenerate and re-energize from physical tiredness.

REM is the sleep stage when we dream. This stage allows a person to recover from psychological fatigue and stress. It follows deep sleep and represents 20% to 25% of total sleep, i.e. nearly 2 hours per night. In REM, the face moves and is expressive. Although the eyelids are closed, the eyes move rapidly under the lids, which indicates intense brain activity that corresponds to dreaming. It is common to wake up suddenly in the morning at the end of a phase of REM sleep.

Sleep Problems

While most of us will have the odd bad night of sleep, there are millions of people who have on-going sleep challenges. These people either accept that they don't sleep well or turn to pills to help. This is often without any real investigation or attempt to understand what factors might be causing poor sleep.

Insomnia is a general term describing difficulty falling asleep and staying asleep. It is the most common sleep problem, with most people suffering at least occasional insomnia, and 10– 15% reporting a chronic condition. Such sleep issues can have myriad different causes, including psychological stress, a sub optimal sleep environment, an inconsistent sleep schedule, or excessive mental or physical stimulation in the hours before bedtime.

Treating insomnia may be through behavioral changes like keeping a more regular sleep schedule, avoiding stimulating activities in the hours before bed, and eliminating or reducing stimulants such as caffeine or sugar. The bedroom environment may be made more conducive to good sleep by using black-out blinds as well as keeping modern distractions such as computers, televisions and back-lit readers out of the bedroom. Tracking down which of these to address in each individual situation may be aided by some of the technologies in this chapter.

A 2010 review of published scientific research suggested that exercise generally improves sleep for most people, and helps sleep disorders such as insomnia. The optimum time to exercise may be 4 to 8 hours before bedtime, though exercise at any time of day is beneficial, with the exception of heavy exercise taken shortly before bedtime, which may disturb sleep. However, there is insufficient evidence to draw detailed conclusions about the relationship between exercise and sleep.

The Impacts of Sleep Deprivation

The potential negative impact of irregular or insufficient sleep has been carefully studied by several academics. A 2014 investigation by the BBC into modern sleep habits saw Scientists from Oxford, Cambridge, Harvard, Manchester and Surrey universities warn that cutting sleep is leading to "serious health problems". They say people and governments need to take the problem seriously as cancer, heart disease, type-2 diabetes, infections and obesity have all been linked to reduced sleep.

A recent New York Times article warned that failing to get enough sleep night after night can compromise your health and may even shorten your life. It also noted that the effects of inadequate sleep can profoundly affect memory, learning, creativity, productivity and emotional stability, as well as your physical health.

According to sleep specialists at the University of Pittsburgh School of Medicine and Western Psychiatric Institute and Clinic, among others, a number of bodily systems are negatively affected by inadequate sleep: the heart, lungs and kidneys; appetite, metabolism and weight control; immune function and disease resistance; sensitivity to pain; reaction time; mood; and brain function. Several studies have linked insufficient sleep to weight gain. Not only do night owls with shortchanged sleep have more time to eat, drink and snack, but levels of the hormone leptin, which tells the brain enough food has been consumed, are lower in the sleep-deprived while levels of ghrelin, which stimulates appetite, are higher. In addition, metabolism slows when one's circadian rhythm and sleep are disrupted; if not counteracted by increased exercise or reduced caloric intake, this slowdown could add up to 10 extra pounds in a year - or to put it another way, if you don't devote enough attention to sleep, it could undo all your good work to lose weight by increasing your exercise or managing your diet.

During sleep, the body produces cytokines, cellular hormones that help fight infections. Thus, short sleepers may be more susceptible to everyday infections like colds and flu. In a study of 153 healthy men and women, Sheldon Cohen and colleagues at Carnegie Mellon University found that those who slept less than seven hours a night were three times as likely to develop cold symptoms when exposed to a cold-causing virus than were people who slept eight or more hours.

As an article in Wired pointed out in February 2015, every year sufferers of sleep apnea—a breathing disorder caused when throat muscles relax and block the airway during sleep—get into car accidents, causing over a thousand deaths. Apnea is linked to obesity, heart disease, diabetes, an additional $3.4 billion in medical costs, and $16 billion in auto collision costs. Even though apnea has telltale signs (loud snoring, daytime fatigue), it goes undiagnosed 75 percent of the time due to the expensive and inconvenient technology traditionally used to diagnose sleep apnea: Polysomnography which requires a medical technician to attach 22 wires to a person's body and monitor them all night long at an average cost of nearly $3,000.

Yet more recent studies have tied sleep closely to our ability to form new memories and recall old ones. Sleep seems to be the time our brains engage in "memory consolidation," which is essentially the process by which short term memories become cemented into long-term memories. Disrupted sleep can impair this process. In general, the study found an inverse relationship between sleep duration and weight gain. So much of our overall well-being is linked - sleep is good for mental well-being, as is exercise and what you eat. Exercise impacts your sleep. Studies show that sleep is the third piece in the trifecta with nutrition and activity for staying fit and maintaining a healthy weight.

Measuring Sleep

If you ask most people how they slept, they will reply with "well" or "badly". We don't tend to ascribe huge detailed descriptions to how we sleep. But as we saw above, whether we're aware of it or not, we all go through phases as we sleep. As with activity, while you may know you don't get enough sleep instinctively, having it drawn out for you in a graph can help focus on the facts and move out of the realm of instinct. It may also illustrate a lack of consistency in your sleep pattern - first off, a record of your bedtime is hard to argue with. A routine is an important part of a good sleep pattern.

Similar to activity and food tracking, starting to improve your sleep can be as simple as awareness, underpinned by graphs and data that you can't kid yourself about. While many people know they tend to stay up later than they should, when presented with the evidence of just how late they stay up, they may change their behavior and pull back their bedtime to give themselves a chance of getting enough sleep.

Choice of Technologies

The plethora of sleep-related consumer technologies that have appeared in the last couple of years ranges from the simple app-based sleep tracker to complete sleep "systems" that try to help you sleep, monitor your sleep and provide advice based on both the quality of your sleep and the physical environment. You can choose from a range of consumer products designed to monitor sleep and related elements, such as heart rate, respiration, motion or even the bedroom's temperature, light levels and noise levels. Whether the devices are strapped to your wrist, chest, mattress or perched on a nightstand, they aim to analyze your sleep cycles and rate their quality.

As with activity trackers we looked at in a previous chapter, there are now all manner of sleep monitoring gadgets. In fact, a number of the activity trackers by day switch to sleep trackers by night. But along with the wrist-worn or clip-on devices, there is a variety of dedicated sleep monitoring technologies that again take a variety of approaches to analyze our sleep without being so invasive as to interfere with it.

When looking to measure sleep and sleep quality, there sensor can be in one or more of the following locations:

- On the person (wrist or clip on)
- On the bed (attached to the pillow, under the sheet or under the mattress)
- Built into the bed itself
- In the phone beside the bed

Sensor solutions exist where you and your partner both want to measure sleep. Obviously wearing individual wrist or clip on solutions allows for personal monitoring, but on-bed sensors also provide separate data for both sides of the bed.

Your choice of sleep technology may well depend on a number of factors:

- Do you feel you have a sleep problem or significant room for improvement in your sleep regime?
- Do you already have an existing activity tracking solution?

- Are you sensitive to wearing a wrist sensor while sleeping?
- Do you want to investigate environmental influences?

As with other technologies we look at in this book, the ones that require the least interaction are the most effective. Sleep trackers that need you to tell them when you're going to sleep depend for their efficacy on the user remembering to press a button (or a sequence of buttons) to enable sleep mode. I'm glad to see recent models adding automatic sensing of sleep to their feature set, but with a little habit, it isn't a big imposition.

The more complex systems not only monitor your sleep but also actively try to help you go to sleep, and provide extremely detailed information. In fact, under the heading of sleep monitoring technologies, solutions are now available to assess the quality of our sleep covering a bewildering number of aspects and influences:

- Time in bed
- Time taken to fall asleep
- Deep Sleep
- Light Sleep
- Snoring
- Breathing
- Heart Rate
- Temperature
- Air Quality
- Light Levels

The most basic level of sleep tracking is keeping a record of when you went to bed, when you fell asleep and when you woke up. This information can at least show patterns of going to bed too late that may prompt a behavioral change. But in order to start getting any more significant insights into the quality of your sleep, you need to start tracking more details.

Sleep Apps

There are plenty of apps available but one of the most popular - downloaded over 1 million times on Android alone is Sleep Better with Runtastic. It claims to help you track your sleep, monitor your dreams, improve your bedtime habits and wake up better. By installing the app and placing your phone next to your pillow, it uses your phone's sensors to monitor your movements as you sleep. Additional diary features enable you to record daily habits, such as caffeine consumption, exercise info, alcohol consumption and stress level, to determine the effects of these variables on your sleep quality, as well as monitoring moon phases.

Activity Trackers

Many of the activity trackers also moonlight as sleep trackers. If you leave them on your wrist (easy in the case of the wrist band style) or move them from your belt to your night wear or put them into a soft wrist holder (in the case of clip-on trackers), then these devices will use your body movement through the night to determine the phases of your sleep cycle and report that back to you. Most also offer some form of smart alarm that will vibrate to wake you during the lightest sleep phase as close as possible the ideal waking time you've set.

Some activity trackers need to be switched into a sleep mode, while others detect your reduction of movement compared to waking hours and automatically switch modes, deducing you've gone to sleep. In their sleep configurations, their accelerometers are more sensitive to small movements that would be of no interest during active daily use. Despite their sensitivity, some sleep experts point to brain waves as the only true measure of sleep stage, with differences in physical movements not being definitive. Makers of activity trackers counter that the amounts of movement they track are a reasonable proxy for sleep stage and provide an acceptable level of accuracy for a convenient consumer product compared to laboratory or clinical results. As I've said repeatedly, I believe that the awareness these products promote and the conversations they enable are more important than their ultimate accuracy.

Sleep Sensors

The next category of tech beyond activity trackers comprises dedicated sleep systems that involve one or more sensors either in the bed or on your nightstand, or a mixture. While I personally can sleep easily with a wrist-worn solution, I know many people prefer to be unencumbered with jewelry while they sleep. In this cases, a contact-free solution is preferable so the sleep tracking device to interfere with sleep comfort!

There are even beds with built-in sleep monitoring technology but I'm going to largely ignore them here for two reasons: I haven't personally tried them so don't feel well placed to comment on them and they are prohibitively expensive for most people who don't have a very deep interest in sleep data.

At the time of writing, these are the main sleep devices/systems available:

- Another example of a startup crowd-funded product rather than from a more traditional manufacturing company, Beddit is an ultra-thin sensor that you stick to your mattress under your sheet at approximately chest height. This device uses ballistocardiography (BCG), a method which uses motion sensing to detect individual heartbeats and breathing rhythm. The associated app measures bed time, awakenings and bed exits, sleep time, sleep latency (the time it takes to fall asleep), resting heart rate, sleep quality and breathing movements, which also analyses if the user is snoring. The sensor uses Bluetooth to connect with the companion app, which offers personalized coaching, a wellness diary, a history of sleep recordings and a social sharing option. Separate Beddit sensors are required for each side of the bed.

- At $249, one of the more expensive domestic devices, the Withings Aura system uses a mattress sensor to monitor body movements, breathing cycles and heart rate, while the bedside device senses ambient environmental factors like noise, light, and temperature. The bedside device also emits light and sound to help users fall asleep or wake up. The program is designed to help relax users as they fall asleep by facilitating the release of the hormone melatonin into the body and help them wake up more easily in the morning. When you're ready to sleep, you simply tap the top of the device and it projects a red light which encourages the production of melatonin. It also offers a range of soothing noises (such as lapping waves) that gradually reduce as you fall asleep. One of the more advanced sleep systems on the market, it tries to tackle the whole sleep cycle, from falling asleep to monitoring the environment when you're asleep to waking you up. Plugging your phone in to it to charge will turn off the wireless elements of your phone too to avoid interruptions, and you can even have it tell your separate smart thermostat (such as the one sold by Nest) to optimize the temperature for sleep. While you only need one bedside unit per bed, additional sensors for under the mattress can be purchased if required.

- The Sense device is another crowdfunded newcomer, this time a small orb-shaped device that sits on a bedside table and tracks the noise, light, humidity, and temperature in the user's bedroom. The device turns green when it senses the room is at an appropriate temperature, light level and noise level. Sense pings a user's app if it finds their room is not at a proper environment for sleeping yet. The system also includes a small clip, called Sleep Pill, that attaches to the user's pillow. After a night of sleep, the Sense app shows user's sleeping patterns detected by the Pill clip as well as environmental data tracked by the bedside device. As with the other bedside solutions, just one unit is required but separate pills facilitate individual tracking.

- S+ is the first consumer sleep product from Resmed who have a long history of producing medical grade sleep devices. Like the Aura it has a bedside unit but it does not have any additional sensor under the sheet (like Beddit), under the Mattress (like Aura) or on the pillow (like Sense). It relies instead on radio waves pointed at the sleeper from the main unit. The $150 non-contact sleep sensor sits within arm's length of your bed and connects to a smartphone and the S+ app. The wireless device monitors breathing patterns, body movements and the bedroom's light, noise and temperature. The app allows users to log the day's stress level, exercise time, caffeine and alcohol intake. In the morning, the app tallies a sleep score based on REM, deep and light sleep levels. A "mind-clear" function records voice or text memos, so nagging thoughts can be put to bed too. S+ differs from the other solutions above in that due to its different approach of not using a sensor in or on the bed, a separate unit is required to track two sleepers in a double bed. It is the only one of the sleep systems I've tried that is designed to be portable - you can put the sensor unit easily in the corner of a suitcase and bring it with you when you travel, whereas it really isn't practical to start installing sensors like Beddit or Aura in a hotel room.

Analysing Sleep Data

While we've seen how activity trackers can quantify the unknown for us (e.g. giving a clear numeric counter of the number of steps we take each day that we probably weren't aware of), sleep tracking is a different ball game. Most people do have a fair idea of how much they sleep - simply counting the time between going to bed and getting up gives you a reasonable idea of the maximum amount of sleep you could have gotten. So what actionable information can these technologies provide:

- Sleep Time
- Environmental Factors
- Personal Factors (see next chapter)

The various devices and their apps are also able to give you some context - if you think you don't get enough sleep for example, you can learn how your sleep pattern compares to people of your own age around the world. The app can remind you what a suggested bedtime would be in order to get the recommended amount of sleep. It also points out patterns - such as that you tend to go to bed late on a Friday.

Apps can also help you draw correlations between events in your day and your sleep. For example if you eat late, exercise late or drink too much caffeine, you may find it harder to sleep. The Jawbone Coffee App monitors the link between sleep and coffee intake during the day. You simply tell it how much coffee you drink (it comes conveniently ready-programmed with the caffeine dosages found in big-name coffee shop sizes) and it uses the sleep tracking feature of your Up wristband to analyze the link between the two.

Most people don't like to be told to go to bed. Maybe it stems from when we were children and constantly fought with our parents to be allowed to stay up later. But just as with resistance to taking more exercise, resistance to placing sufficient importance on getting enough sleep and enough good quality sleep may come back to haunt us.

If you do suffer from a serious sleep issue such as sleep apnea, mobile technologies may also offer hope - the University of Washington for example is developing an app to offer medical-grade diagnosis the equivalent of thousands of dollars of polysomnography.

As we've now pretty much covered off the area of monitoring your sleep, the last topic I want to discuss in this section is about what technology may affect you just before you fall asleep and just as you wake up.

Getting to Sleep: Lights & Tech Out

In the past 50 years, there has been a decline in average sleep duration and quality as artificial lighting expands virtually globally and people have more gadgets and media outlets vying for their time than ever.

Most of this book is quite positive and optimistic about the impact that mobile phones can and will have on our well-being when used correctly and with the right amount of common sense. However, there is an area where they have a demonstrable and immediate negative impact - preventing us going to sleep. For the millions of people who stare at their phone or tablet screens while in bed, it's harder to go to sleep. This is not just because it keeps our minds active but the phones affect us chemically. The bright screens, and specifically the blueish light they emit interfere with the body's production of its sleep inducing chemical, melatonin.

Prof Charles Czeisler, from Harvard University recently told a BBC report on Sleep: "It's a big concern that we're being exposed to much more light, sleeping less and, as a consequence, may suffer from many chronic diseases." The modern house and bedroom has multiple sources of high intensity light - energy efficient light bulbs as well as smartphones, tablets and computers have high levels of light in the blue end of the spectrum which is "right in the sweet spot" for disrupting the body clock. "Light exposure, especially short wavelength blue-ish light in the evening, will reset our circadian rhythms to a later hour, postponing the release of the sleep-promoting hormone melatonin and making it more difficult for us to get up in the morning."

Many people use their phone or tablet in bed and actually make it an important part of their end of day relaxation ritual to catch up on social networks, the last bit of work or a favorite TV show. Inadvertently stimulating their body via these bright screens, they may find it interesting to compare the time taken to go to sleep on nights they don't use back-lit screens before trying to sleep. But for those who can't abide the thought of losing these last few minutes of screen time before sleep, at least there are apps that promise to help a little: Twilight for example is an app that reduces the blue-intensity of your screen, dimming it to a level that is less likely to inhibit your melatonin production.

The End of Sleep

Fittingly enough as we come to the end of the sleep discussion, it's time to discuss waking. Many sleep trackers include intelligent alarm functionality. This feature aims to wake you at the optimum time in your sleep cycle, when you are in a light sleep. It's easier to rouse you from a light sleep, and leaves you feeling less groggy. Of course you may be in a deep cycle at the time you've specified for your alarm, getting your day off to a bad start. Smart alarms allow you to specify a window of time during which you want to be woken rather than just a specific time. Let's say you set an alarm for 7.30 but with a 20 minute window. If at 7.15, the device detects you're in a light sleep cycle, it will wake you then - earlier than your 7.30 alarm but with the benefits of not trying to pull you out of a deep sleep.

Sleep Better in a Smart Home ?

If you decide to investigate your sleep with some of the more advanced devices, you may conclude, with the insights from your technology, that environmental factors are contributing to your getting sub-optimal sleep.

The Aura system mentioned earlier tracks the light and sound levels in the room. In the next chapter we'll look at some of the environmental sensors available for your home today, which may contribute additional information to your sleep analysis if used in the bedroom as well as throughout your house. Although not strictly a sleep-related tool, room/environment sensors such as those made by Netatmo measure multiple factors that could impact on sleep.

Although integration of health and well-being devices with a smart home is beyond the scope of this book, there will inevitably be deeper relationships between the gadgets we're surrounded with and they will start to swap information. You can take things a stage further by linking waking time not only to the temperature but also to a WiFi enabled coffee maker so there's a fresh cup of coffee waiting for you as soon as you wake up - now all we need is a robot to deliver it!

But leaving aside the convenience of waking to a piping fresh cup of coffee, there are potentially serious benefits of integrating your sleep information with smart home technology that regulates your environment. For example, if your chosen sleep sensor monitors say temperature and notices that you sleep better at a certain temperature, you can have it regulate the temperature automatically using either heating or cooling to restore the equilibrium. If the CO_2 level in the bedroom is too high, you can have a fan come on to stir the air and reduce it.

Learning about your sleep habits can help you improve them - for example, if you find out that you're only getting 5 hours of sleep per night, maybe it's time to start heading to bed earlier or waking up later. Improving your sleep habits can ultimately improve your life, and requires less effort than exercise and less willpower than dieting. Having now looked at your exercise, food intake and sleep habits, the next area of well-being we'll turn to in Chapter 7 is your mental well-being.

Chapter 7:
The Brain, Stress & Mood

"Mens sana in corpore sano."
(A healthy mind in a healthy body)

- Roman poet Juvenal in the first century.

Despite there having been a nearly endless succession of various fitness crazes over the years and the concept of dieting which dates back over 100 years, the amount of attention we pay to the most complex organ in our bodies remains relatively limited. Brain health is not a very common topic - perhaps partly because we know so little about it and partly because in a frequently superficial world, it's hidden - while you can easily see people who are overweight or people who are exercising, it's much harder to see people who look after their brain or don't.

Although in terms of outright size, it's only the third largest organ in the human body (behind the skin and the liver), the brain is easily the most complex. Made up of an average of over 80 billion neurons, the brain exerts control over the other organs of the body both by managing patterns of muscle activity and by managing the secretion of a wide variety of chemicals we know collectively as hormones via a network of glands.

When talking about health care, many people are referring only to their physical health. The area of mental health and well-being doesn't yet receive significant popular attention. Yet the brain is such a complex organ that we understand even less about its operation than we do much of the rest of the human body. However, its influence on our well-being is massive. It is of course as we've noted harder to observe and somewhat less accessible than the rest of our body, but that is no reason why we shouldn't look to safeguard and even improve its well-being.

While many people visit a physician on a regular basis, few visit a mental health professional. And while 30% of people do profess to pay some level of attention to their exercise levels or their caloric intake, a negligible number are particularly aware of their mental state, measure it, or take any proactive steps to improve it.

Accessing the Brain

Even though, before the advent of the revolution we describe in this book, we may not have historically had access to the various diagnostic devices that medical professionals have, most of us are somewhat familiar with the blood pressure monitor or blood oxygen monitor in the doctor's surgery, as well as other tools of the trade such as sample sticks. These are now all readily available to individuals with smartphones for self-use and interpretation as we've seen but while you can ask a group of people to name tools related to their physical health, how many would be able to name devices that serve to monitor mental well-being via scanners or sensors?

The tools of the trade for brain evaluation are much more limited than those available for the rest of the body. Technological advances in recent decades have brought unprecedented insights into brain composition, function and activity via developments such as Functional Magnetic Resonance Imaging (fMRI) which measures the blood flow in the brain and Electroencephalography (EEGs) which measures electrical activity. Combined with other clinical-scale machines such as Positron Emission Tomography/Computed Tomography (PET/CT), neuroscience has made great strides in unlocking the mysteries of our so-called Grey Matter (which is actually more pink/beige than grey).

Even though the aforementioned complex diagnostic tools such as MRIs are room-sized or involve radiation (PET/CT), and likely to remain the preserve of professionals and researchers for many years to come, there are still areas of neuroscience that are not immune to the advance of the smartphone and there is now a multitude of smartphone-centric devices that can assist in monitoring your brain and the physical manifestations of stress.

I'll look in this chapter at four areas where mobile technology and related accessories can help with your understanding of your mental state including:

- Stress
- Mindfulness
- Breathing
- Brain Training

Stress

Stress has worked its way into the vernacular these days as a general descriptor for people feeling anything from tired to borderline clinically depressed. Abused a bit like the word shock (which also has a very specific medical meaning), stress in its strictest sense means the response of the body to an external stimulus or challenge.

Physiological stress describes a wide range of physical responses that occur as a direct effect of a stressor causing a disruption in the homeostasis (the relatively stable internal environment) of the body. In the event of disruption of either psychological or physical equilibrium, the brain (specifically an area of the brain known as the amygdala) triggers a response by stimulating various bodily subsystems including the nervous, endocrine (glands), and immune systems. The reaction of these systems causes a number of physical changes that have both short- and long-term effects on the body. Their first impact is to increase our heart rate and blood pressure, as well as our breathing. This allows us to transport oxygen to our muscles quickly so we can "act fast", but this heightened state is a short-term condition.

Although only studied in depth as a medical field in the last century, stress is nothing new and your body is equipped to deal with a certain amount of it. Various hormones, such as adrenaline and norepinephrine help you deal with high-stress situations and are intended for short-term effects to help you escape danger. The body's other main stress-combatant is cortisol, which is slower-acting than the other two, but still not meant for sustained use. However, if you are under persistent stress, then you may have elevated cortisol levels on an on-going basis which affects your immune system and potentially your bones, as well as promoting bad eating habits by making you crave fatty foods. A bit of stress in short doses is useful in improving our memory and enhancing performance. However, too much, too regularly, is extremely damaging to our mental and physical well-being. It can lead to stomach ulcers, heart problems, illnesses, lowered libido and many more ailments.

Reducing stress, then, may seem like an instinctively good idea but it's important to understand the role stress plays in our body - positive when it's needed but potentially harmful if it continues beyond its useful time. When we are threatened, our bodies initiate a stress response, releasing hormones, increasing heart rate, and supplying sugar to our muscles. It also shuts down non-essential systems (such as digestion) that might divert energy which could inhibit a fight or flight response. These changes were the difference between life and death for cavemen. Fast forward to today and our minds have evolved a lot faster than our bodies. Our bodies still respond to things that threaten us, but the "stressors" that our minds perceive as threats are often no longer imminent physical threats as they were for our ancestors.

Much research has shown the negative effect acute stress has on the immune system, which starts to produce natural defensive cells as if the body was fighting infection. Chronic or prolonged stress may cause various physical manifestations and take a more significant toll on the body than acute stress does. It can raise blood pressure, increase the risk of heart attack and stroke, increase vulnerability to anxiety and depression, contribute to infertility, and hasten the aging process. While responses to acute stressors typically do not impose a health burden on young, healthy individuals, chronic stress in older or unhealthy individuals may have long-term effects detrimental to health.

The Costs of Stress

Today's fast paced world makes it difficult to find time to de-stress. Moreover, while many people feel stressed they find it hard to quantify or know if they are succeeding in reducing it. We may not be aware of it, but virtually everyone has personal experience of stress. We all know that too much stress is bad for us. It is a global problem with huge economic and societal cost. According to the Anxiety and Depression Association of America, anxiety disorders are the most common mental illness in the US - affecting 40 million adults. The World Health Organization says it costs businesses in the US $300bn a year and the UK's Health and Safety Executive recently reported that over 11.4 million days were lost due to work-related stress in 2013/2014 in the UK. So once again, if technology can help to identify the problem and increase awareness and management of it, the potential benefits are enormous.

In a 2012 survey, 20% of Americans said they were experiencing extreme levels of stress. And while 64% said that it is "extremely important or very important to manage stress", only 37% felt they were actually doing an excellent or very good job at managing theirs. A UK survey of over 2,000 people found that 80% think "life's moving too fast and that the number of things we have to do and worry about these days is a major cause of stress, unhappiness and illness". Over 50% said they had "difficulty relaxing or switching off", and that they couldn't stop thinking about "things they've got to do". Mobile phones are often blamed for exacerbating this trend, and without a doubt there are times when people could benefit from disconnecting from an always-on life that blurs the boundaries between work and personal life. But if used appropriately, smartphones can be a major contributor to reducing stress.

From the Mental to the Physical

Although loosely applied to a range of symptoms or sometimes the absence of symptoms not always immediately apparent, stress does have physical manifestations:

- Heart Rate
- Skin Temperature
- Skin Reactions
- Breathing rate

Heart Rate Variability (HRV)

We've already covered heart rate in the chapter on vital signs so you're familiar with the tools available to monitor heart rate and the importance of heart rate zones for exercise and training, but in this context, we're more interested in heart rate variability.

HRV indicates the fluctuations of heart rate around an average. An average heart rate of 60 beats per minute (bpm) does not mean that the interval between successive heartbeats would be exactly 1.0 sec, instead they may fluctuate/vary from 0.5 sec up to 2.0 sec. Other factors that affect HRV are age, genetics, body position, time of day, and health status. During exercise, HRV decreases as heart rate and exercise intensity increase. HRV also decreases during periods of mental stress.

Bio Feedback

Along with HRV, the most common form of stress measurement is via bio feedback. Biofeedback-assisted relaxation training (BART) is a proven, effective protocol for stress reduction. It trains people to reduce stress by using biosignals from their own bodies. Electrodermal Activity (EDA) – the electrical activity of the sweat glands in the skin – is a well-established biosignal for emotional stress. Our levels of stress fluctuate continuously – significant changes happen in fractions of a second; and with the fluctuation, the electrical properties of our skin change. The skin at our fingertips acts as a particularly sensitive indicator. When we are stressed, we sweat – resulting in our skin's conductance of electricity improving briefly. Fingertips are the best place to measure the skin's response to stress. This is sometimes also referred to as galvanic skin response (GSR). And for anyone who thought GSR stood for Gun Shot Residue, your stress may be due to watching too many forensic police shows - it might be time to give NCIS a break!

The only popular phones with built in stress measuring capabilities are the Samsung S5/S6 and the Samsung Galaxy Note 4 via the included S-Health app and the heart rate sensor on the back of the device. Based on HRV, it rates your stress levels from low to high. The Microsoft Band and the HealBe GoBe are two wrist-worn devices mentioned earlier that also report your stress levels.

One example of a dedicated consumer biofeedback device is the PIP - this small device (approximately the size of a small key fob) is held between your thumb and forefinger to detect electrodermal activity. It sends the data to an app on your smartphone via Bluetooth to help you measure and ideally learn to manage stress. It's very easy to use - just hold the device and follow the prompts on your screen. The gold-plated sensors measure your GSR at the rate of 8 times per second and the device comes with a selection of apps that represent your stress levels as mini games. The more you can train yourself to relax and lower your stress, the better you perform in the games.

Its small size means it's easy to keep with you and use when you have a few spare minutes or feel the need to manage your stress levels. The app records your progress over time and supports multiple profiles, so you can share it with family or friends. At $180, it's one of the more expensive and niche gadgets covered here, but as with most examples, it may be of particular benefit to a select group. But while measuring your stress levels is a start, there is more help available from your mobile to develop relaxation techniques and abilities.

Another example is the Spire clip-on activity and stress tracker that sits on your belt or bra and monitors your respiration and movements rather than your heart rate or heart rate variability. Even more discrete than the PIP as you wear it rather than hold it, it reports on your entire day's stress levels categorized into calm, focused and tense; and also features reminders on your phone should you exhibit too much tension, exhorting you to take break.

Meditation & Mindfulness

Meditation as a practice can evoke quite strong reactions and preconceptions. As with many of the topics in this book, it has supporters and detractors, cynics and zealots. As always, my purpose in discussing it here is to ensure that people are aware of it and consider its potential relevance, assess if it may have any benefits and potentially try it with the aid of mobile technology. Although an ancient art, meditation has undergone a modern revolution with the advent of mobile technology that has made it more accessible to a wider audience than ever before.

Mindfulness is a very simple form of meditation that was little known in the West until quite recently. In this context mindfulness is defined as moment-by-moment awareness of thoughts, feelings, bodily sensations, and surrounding environment, characterized mainly by "acceptance" - attention to thoughts and feelings without judging whether they are right or wrong. Mindfulness focuses the human brain on what is being sensed at each moment, instead of on its normal occupation with assessing the past or considering future scenarios. A typical meditation consists of focusing your full attention on your breath as it flows in and out of your body. Focusing on each breath in this way allows you to observe your thoughts as they arise in your mind and, little by little, to let go of struggling with them. You come to realize that thoughts come and go of their own accord. Mindfulness is about observation without criticism; when unhappiness or stress hover overhead, rather than taking it all personally, you learn to treat them as if they were black clouds in the sky, and to observe them with friendly curiosity as they drift past.

Many myths attend meditation so it's worth clarifying how the popular modern form should be assessed:

- You don't have to sit cross-legged on the floor (though you can if you want to). Most people sit on chairs, but you can also practice bringing mindful awareness to whatever you are doing, on buses, trains or while walking to work.
- Mindfulness practice does not take a lot of time, although some patience and persistence are required. Popular apps offer sessions from 5 to 30 or 40 minutes at a time.

It is somewhat ironic when you have examples of ancient wisdom being made more accessible via modern technology. The monks who developed mindfulness concepts over 2500 years ago can hardly have imaged a future where busy commuters would be sat on a bus or a train, earphones in, with meditation exercises being run by their phones.

Much scientific study in recent years is available to back-up claims of wide-ranging benefits from Meditation - making it firmly evidence-based. In one well known study, senior author Sara Lazar (of the Massachusetts General Hospital Psychiatric Neuroimaging Research Program and a Harvard Medical School instructor in psychology) noted "This study demonstrates that changes in brain structure may underlie some of these reported improvements and that people are not just feeling better because they are spending time relaxing. We took people who'd never meditated before, and put one group through an eight-week mindfulness-based stress reduction program where subjects took a weekly class. They were given a recording and told to practice 40 minutes a day at home. We found differences in brain volume after eight weeks in five different regions in the brains of the two groups. In the group that learned meditation, we found thickening in four regions, including the amygdala, the fight or flight part of the brain which is important for anxiety, fear and stress in general. That area got smaller in the group that went through the mindfulness-based stress reduction program. The change in the amygdala was also correlated to a reduction in stress levels. Similarly, researchers from Harvard University discovered corresponding changes in the physical structure of the brain with a similar meditation course; there was a lower density of neurons in the amygdala and greater density of neurons in areas involved in emotional control - evidence that meditation served as a realistic and maintainable stress management technique."

Mindfulness Apps

There is a variety of mindfulness apps available but there seem to be a few clear leaders in the field - Headspace and Calm which have over 1,000,000 downloads each. But before we look at the kind of features these apps deliver in more detail, it's worth highlighting the specific benefits of using mobile technologies to support mediation:

- Always available
- Reminders to help you create the habit
- Personal use requires no additional equipment - most people have earphones

- Unobtrusive with no accessory or additional charging required
- No cost to try

Headspace is a highly polished and professional looking app; I had come across it when looking at the emerging space of health-related apps. But it was when in conversation with a professional psychologist who recommended Headspace that I was intrigued enough to evaluate it more comprehensively.

- The Headspace app is available for a free trial, with paid content available within the app that covers a wide range of topics and includes different duration meditation sessions and different levels of guidance, where the facilitator offers varying degrees of help as you listen. It also features emergency sessions if you find yourself under stress and allows you to add Buddies so you can share progress updates with a selection of friends. It also uses "Streaks" to motivate continued use with little badges and offers of discounts for consecutive days. Headspace also claims benefits for creativity, focus, anxiety, self-esteem and relationships. Lots of facts and figures, claims and evidence is presented on the Headspace website but my advice would be to try it for yourself before deciding if you want to subscribe.

- The Calm app offers 7-day and 21-day guided meditation sessions of varying daily durations to fit your schedule. It offers calming photos with background sounds and music tracks to help you relax. Premium topics include guided meditations for focus, creativity, energy, confidence, and sleep.

Mindfulness is just like exercise. It's a form of mental exercise, really. And just as exercise increases health, helps us handle stress better and promotes longevity, meditation purports to confer some of those same benefits. But, just like exercise, it can't cure everything. So the idea is, it's useful as an adjunct therapy. And it doesn't work for everybody. While Mindfulness depends on the exercises that can be easily listened to from phone, deeper investigation of your mind and stress can be undertaken with the addition of some sensors. Not yet typically built in to phones, there are some peripherals designed to monitor external signs of stress.

Brain Waves

Let's take a slightly closer look at the center of your nervous system and the organ we've mentioned several times in connection with stress - the brain. Despite the 90s being declared the decade of the brain and the huge advances in neuroscience in recent years, humans still know relatively little about the intricacies of the brain. However, advances in imaging and monitoring tools will continue to see our knowledge about our knowledge center continue to improve.

The most commonly used form of brain activity tracking is Electroencephalography (EEG) - the measurement of electric activity produced by the brain. The neurons in our brain communicate by sending small electrical impulses to each other. When a large number of neurons fire at the same time they create a change in the electric field we can measure from outside the head. When neurons fire, we can calculate the strength of certain frequencies and correlate to general states of mind. These brain waves travel at different frequencies and measuring these can identify if your mind is calm and focused, and when it is wandering. Brain signals are very weak and they can range from 1 microvolt to 300 microvolts (a microvolt is one millionth of a volt). Some perspective: an AA battery is 1.5 million times stronger than the weakest brain signal.

EEG is a non-invasive (thankfully when we're talking about monitoring brain activity!) way to record the brain's spontaneous electrical activity over a period of time. Its origins date back nearly 100 years but it's only in the last couple of years that the notion of personal EEG devices has been possible. While a clinical EEG (such as used to diagnose epilepsy) takes about 30 minutes, the domestic versions used to identify restful brain states typically take only a few minutes. They provide a relatively superficial view of the brain's state and activity but represent a first step in awareness, measurement and understanding.

A wearable device of interest for those wanting to better understand their brain is a headband called Muse from a Canadian company. With it, a person can track their brain activity in real time on a smartphone or tablet, and practice focused attention. It's a clinical grade EEG, looking like a slightly oddly designed set of earphones (all the odder because the sit behind your ear not on your ear); the MUSE headband measures your brainwaves. Where Muse can help, compared to simple apps that guide you through your meditation, is that it graphically illustrates the changes in your brain patterns as you become more relaxed or tense.

We've already seen evidence that the focused-attention and mindfulness exercises cause the brain to change itself, but the gamification approach makes this process more motivating as you see the impact over time and can correlate readings with events. The Muse app starts you with 3 minute sessions and rewards you for your achievements, attempting to form the habit of regular exercise. If you want to build your strength and endurance, you can do repetitive physical exercises like running or walking. Similarly, to improve a specific cognitive skill like attention, you can perform a repetitive mental exercise and reap the benefits over time.

When you learn how to manage and respond to emotionally charged thoughts, it improves not only your focus, it also improves your self-awareness – the key facet of emotional intelligence. This can lead to decreased emotional reactivity, and increased positive emotion.

Brain Training

While mediation and tracking your brain's activity is closely tied to managing stress, mobile technology is also invading other neural disciplines and exploiting our growing knowledge about the brain to help us improve its well-being and its performance. For centuries, scientists believed that most brain development occurred in the first few years of life — that by adulthood the brain was largely immutable. But over the past two decades, studies on animals and humans have found that the brain continues to form new neural connections throughout life.

The brain is organized in functional networks that include millions of brain cells called neurons. The connections between the brain cells that create these networks are changed by the things a person does or experiences. This is called neuroplasticity. MRI scans show how the structure of the brain changes if you practice something repeatedly.

The first mass-market brain training product was actually the Nintendo DS handheld games console. It was developed in conjunction with Japanese neuroscientist Dr Ryuta Kawashima who was already well known in academic circles for his work involving mapping the regions of the brain which control emotion, language, memorization, and cognition. He rose to widespread fame with the publication of his book - Train Your Brain: 60 Days to a Better Brain. It sold more than two-and-a-half million copies, led to a series of other books and piqued the interest of Nintendo, which turned his program into a game, which itself sold 19 million copies. This casual game made it fun to train your brain - quite a feat given that many people cease to use many aspects of their brain when they leave school....

Once we leave school, we tend to stop any structured attempts at developing brain-power and frequently lapse into routines where new learnings or challenges are rare. We may receive some ongoing job-related training in how to achieve a task, but training in abstract or generic brain skills is rare. But brain training can help you develop new skills as well as protect the skills you already have. While there is no proven link that it can stave off dementia yet, I for one would rather spend 10 minutes a day on these exercises if there's any chance of prolonging my mental performance.

While the Nintendo DS brought brain training exercises to popular attention, not everyone had the device. It was primarily aimed at children and although portable it was not something most adults were going to carry around on a daily basis, just to train their brains. But the meteoric rise of the smartphone since then which has given greater power to virtually every pocket brings us products like Peak and Lumosity. These apps not only offer the user challenging games but add the management, notification and competitive framework as well as frequent updates that make these games compelling and more accessible than ever.

- Lumosity is perhaps the best known of the brain-game websites, with 70 million subscribers in 180 countries. Its range of online games are intended to improve our short and long term memory, flexibility, attention and focus. Designed by neuroscientists, the app offers personalized combinations from over 40 games, complete with global leaderboards.

- Claiming to be both fun and neuroscience-based, Peak is a brain training app intended to track and improve cognitive performance. It includes over 20 mini games across different categories (memory, focus, language, mental agility or problem solving) that are presented in personalized daily workouts. After sessions, it provides In-depth performance tracking with insights including personal and comparative brain maps, data visualizations and per-category graphing (memory, focus, language, mental agility or problem solving).

Does It Work?

While there is no real risk to participating in the many unproven brain-training games available online and through smartphones, experts say, consumers should know that the scientific jury is still out on whether they are really boosting brain health or just paying hundreds of dollars to get better at a game. Questions remain as to whether an intervention that challenges the brain — a puzzle, studying a new language or improving skill on a video game — can really raise intelligence or stave off normal memory loss. Proponents of brain training point to sites like www.cognitivetrainingdata.org/studies-cognitive-training-benefits/ which has over 100 peer-reviewed top-quality scientific research papers reporting studies in which brain training did work. My advice is try it for yourself, see if you enjoy it and see if you feel any better.

In case you're worried that exercising your brain will cause it to increase in size and weight and undo all the good work you've undertaken on the back of the previous chapters, fear not! The average human brain weighs in at about 1.5kg so it's not a significant factor in the number on your scales - in fact only about 2% of total body weight. It does however consume about 20% of your body's energy.

While physical well-being has been taken with increasing seriousness - see the number of gyms, joggers and health food shops, mental wellbeing is something that is rarely talked about. While Yoga and Meditation use has grown, there is little evidence of significant focus on training this vital organ. Since it doesn't require large specialized machinery or changing facilities, there are no gyms for your brain but there are lots of tools to help you better understand it and care for it.

Mood Tracking

Mood tracking is also possible using your mobile. We all have off days where we're in bad humour but rarely do we record it and try to understand any causes. Oftentimes we may not even be aware we're in a bad mood until someone asks us what's wrong. By tracking your mood, and being forced to ask yourself each day to rate your mood, you can become more aware of it, and the factors that influence it.

- Each evening at 9pm my phone reminds me to rate my mood for the day, on a scale of 1 to 5. Using an app called Exist, I can review trends in my mood as well as correlate variations to other factors such as sleep, activity or food. It also demonstrates any correlations to events, weather or even social media activity or inactivity as an influencer of my mood rating.

- Pacifica is an app intended to help tackle stress and anxiety. It is based on Cognitive Behavioral Therapy (CBT), a common psychotherapeutic technique that focuses on identifying, understanding, and changing thinking and behavior patterns. The app encourages you to record your daily mood and associated feelings, as well as your thoughts in a daily audio reflection. You are then asked to listen back to your reflection objectively and categorize positive or negative thoughts before re-recording your reflection. It also provides meditations and experiments for you to try each day and further tracking features include sleep, exercise, diet, hobbies, time spent with people or pets and time spent outdoors.

- The 5 Min Journal app is described as a "toothbrush for the mind". Hopefully they are speaking figuratively, the app prompts you each morning and evening to input things you are grateful for, items you would like to achieve today and affirmations. It also allows you to record photos of positive events and provides daily inspiring quotes, all of which is aimed at creating and maintaining positive thinking patterns.

Apps for Mental Conditions

There is an increasing number of apps targeting support for specific mental conditions. Most are in quite early stages but may be of interest to people dealing with these conditions in their families.

Dementia

When the brain starts to fail, one of the forms this can take is dementia. Here too, companies are starting to investigate how the mobile phone can help in this sensitive area. One example of this is called Backup Memory - an app to prompt people to recall relationships. This provides patients with reminders of people who come to visit them. The app is installed on the sufferer's phone and on the phones of family/visitors. When a visitor is detected, the patient's phone will notify them and display photos of their relationship with that person to help jog their memory and visually stimulate them.

Bipolar

Developers in the University of Michigan are working on an app called Priori that aims to **predict** bipolar episodes before they occur by recording a patient's voice during phone calls, listening for changes in speech patterns, such as speed, that might indicate the onset of a depressive or manic episode. Doctors or caregivers can receive alerts when intervention is deemed advisable by the app.

Lifestyle Choices for Mental Well-Being

Emphasizing the interrelated nature of topics in this book, aside from staying sharp using brain training apps like Peak or Luminosity mentioned above, there are several lifestyle choices you can make to maintain better brain health.

Diet

If you're already maintaining a healthy diet, watching your cholesterol intake and avoiding bad fats, then you are partway there. Current research indicates that a diet low in saturated fats and high in omega-3, vitamin E and lutein can protect brain cells and build good brain health.

Physical Health

Maintaining good physical health is closely linked to brain health. Exercise keeps cholesterol levels in check and maintains good blood flow to the body and brain, stimulating brain plasticity by encouraging growth of new connections between cells. Ensuring you have a regular sleep pattern is also an important aspect of maintaining good brain health.

Social Engagement

It is believed that regular social interaction is a key part to maintaining good brain health. One study showed that men and women with the most social interaction within their community had less than half the rate of memory loss compared to those with the least social engagement. So remember to use your phone to set up social events but don't forget to engage in people activities and not lose all your social time to Netflix or Candy Crush!

Conclusion

The brain remains elusive in terms of our understanding and ability to manipulate it. Most people know that eating affects their weight, and exercise can build muscles, but few know how to manage or improve their brain. Looking after it and developing it are worthy pursuits. It's harder than physical exercise. It's easy to see the outcome of physical training. Anyone who puts in the effort will see the return visibly - either reduced weight, more toned muscles or just increased fitness evident in the small things like being able to climb stairs without being out of breath. Mental exercise doesn't come with such obvious progress but that doesn't mean it's not equally important. While it is less likely to kill us than physical challenges, the personal and societal impacts of mental health are enormous and should be more than enough reason for us to pay our brains a little more attention.

Chapter 8: There's Something For Everyone

For people who are already living a healthy lifestyle with their BASIC monitoring (Brain, Activity, Sleep, Intake & Cardiovascular) under control, the benefits available from the explosion of mobile technologies to enhance well-being are perhaps less dramatic. But that is not to say that tech entrepreneurs haven't dreamt up a range of devices that may still appeal to people for whom other solutions are not relevant and these can still address conditions of major significance to particular individuals.

While many of the advances outlined earlier are quite broad in their applicability, there is a number of more narrowly focused devices that offer very specific solutions. These may not be at the generic lifesaving level of earlier chapters, but they may still make a personally significant improvement to quality of life, or save money. In this section, I'll take a look at solutions designed to tackle some less commonly discussed well-being areas:

- Environment
- Sunlight & Skincare
- Optical Health
- Posture
- Oral Health
- Aural Health
- Vitamins & Minerals
- Medicinal Adherence
- Niche Solutions

Environment

Our environment, through exposure to things like radiation, air pollution, pollen and pesticide in food has a profound impact on our medical essence. Sensors are now becoming available that can quantify and track these exposures.

- Dr. Eric Topol

Large scale environmental issues have been in the news for a significant portion of the last few decades. Global figures from Al Gore to Pope Francis have tackled the issue via movies, lobbying and even a papal encyclical. The emergence of the "green" movement has seen massive change in policies on the burning of fossil fuels, the reduction in CFCs and a focus on preserving rainforests. But regardless of the debates about global warming, climate change and its severity, there has been an unquestionable advance in the understanding of chemical changes in our environment and how they affect us. According to the World Health Organization, air pollution is the world's largest single environmental health risk. Every year, around 7 million people die as a result of air pollution exposure – which is approximately 1 in 8 of total global deaths (WHO, March 2014).

On a more macro level, the impacts of local climate on health have also come to the fore. In particular asthma sufferers are now more likely to monitor air quality information and such information is readily available in many cities who have deployed grids of sensors. Yet given that by definition we spend all our time surrounded by our environment, we tend to know very little about it. We don't generally know how the air quality in our office compares to that in our homes or our cars, nor do we know give much thought to the unseen pollutants that surround us to a greater or lesser extent.

As with many of the medical symptoms we've discussed in this book along with ways to surface awareness of them, our environment is frequently hidden, invisible or ignored, with the exception of obvious pollution like smog. Few people give significant consideration to the real quality of the environment in their homes as long as there is nothing obviously unpleasant.

Whilst it is huge progress that we are increasingly monitoring our bodies, what we put in the them, and how much we exercise, all of these activities ignore another crucial actor upon our well-being - the environment around us. There has long been a recognition in medical circles that environment plays a big part in the human condition. By now you won't be surprised to hear that there is a wide variety of technology-based solutions available to plug any gap in our knowledge and provide both advice and potential remedies based on our individual situation and exposure to atmospheric actors.

What to Measure

The starting point for environmental monitoring is the recording of metrics that are familiar sounding to us - temperature, humidity, pressure are baseline measures that have limited health impacts in most cases unless they are hugely. Devices to deliver these numbers to your mobile start from as little as $40 - an example being the Blucub, a device no bigger than a cubic inch that measures the temperature, noise level and relative humidity in a room. Apart from the influence on sleep mentioned earlier or very extreme cases, managing your domestic temperature is more likely to save you money or help to save the planet than contribute directly to your own well-being. Not surprisingly, your phone could play a decisive role here too with products like the Nest smart thermostat now installed in over 2.5 million US homes and claiming to deliver significant savings by improving temperature regulation.

Air Quality

The next more sophisticated category of sensors starts with products that measure air quality. Carbon monoxide sensors are already widely available and public health campaigns have educated people about the health hazard this colorless, odorless gas poses, particularly in poorly ventilated rooms or where there may be malfunctioning exhausts for boilers. Smart smoke alarms such as the Nest Protect notify your phone via WiFi if it detects CO as well as performing its duties as a smoke alarm.

An example of a mobile-centric device that measures your home environment is the Netatmo weather station which in its basic form consists of an indoor and outdoor module - small cylinders that monitor environmental quality back to your phone. Billed as an urban weather station, these are a far cry from the Stevenson Screen weather monitoring stations that your high school geography teacher used to talk about. These small cylinders have the ability to monitor CO_2, temperature, pollution, noise, humidity, rainfall, as well as alert you to weather forecast events of concern. The sensors track indoor CO_2 level, as well as the noise level, and combine it with temperature to discern a comfort index. You can turn this kind of information into something actionable by for example setting a rule that if the CO_2 level in a room exceeds a certain threshold, you can use a WiFi controlled fan to turn on and circulate the air to freshen things up. The outdoor pollutant information the app reports may be of particular interest to asthmatics or people with other respiratory issues who can base their excursion plans on such readings.

Each year more than 4 million people die from indoor air pollution. People spend on average between 70% and 90% of their time indoors, but unfortunately, indoor air is frequently far more polluted than outdoor air - in fact, indoor air pollution can be ten times as bad as outdoor pollution and can cause headaches, allergies, asthma, and memory loss.

What's In The Air?

There is a multitude of gases and vapors in what we think of as fresh air. CO2 - Carbon dioxide content in fresh air is normally around 400 parts per million (ppm). Prolonged exposure to levels above that may lead to drowsiness or headaches. Along with familiar gases such as CO2, air also contains Volatile Organic Compounds (VOC) - that may sound fairly nasty but VOCs are numerous, varied, and ubiquitous. These vapors include both human-made and naturally occurring chemical compounds and there are thousands of them. Although many countries have standards in place that regulate acceptable levels of VOC in domestic and commercial settings, awareness of them is not generally very high.

Along with the vapors, the air is also replete with atmospheric particulate matter (PM). Unseen in the air around us, there are millions of these particles of varying sizes and origins, which may have an impact on our bodies, especially those people with sensitive lungs. Particulates are the deadliest form of air pollution, due to their ability to penetrate deep into the lungs and blood streams owing to their small size. As with VOCs, particulates can occur naturally, (originating from volcanoes, dust storms, forest fires and sea spray) or due to human activities, such as the burning of fossil fuels in vehicles, power plants and various industrial processes.

Particulate matter is classified according to its size and its presence measured in micrograms (μg)/m^3. The size of particle is the main determinant of how deep into the respiratory tract it will travel when inhaled. Larger particles are generally filtered in the nose and throat but particulate matter smaller than about 10 micrometers, referred to as PM$_{10}$, can travel to the lungs. Still smaller particles (less than 2.5 micrometers), known as PM$_{2.5}$, penetrate further into the lung and even onwards into the circulatory system.

According to the WHO Global Burden of Disease report, PM pollution is estimated to contribute to some 3.22 million deaths globally, while the 2014 study European Study of Cohorts for Air Pollution Effects (ESCAPE) with 100,166 participants, cited an increase in estimated annual exposure to $PM_{2.5}$ of just 5 µg/m^3 was linked with a 13% increased risk of heart attacks. A 2011 study concluded that traffic exhaust is the single most serious preventable cause of heart attack in the general public, the cause of 7.4% of all attacks. The effects of inhaling particulate matter that have been widely researched and include asthma, some lung cancer, cardiovascular disease, respiratory diseases, and premature death.

As yet, there are no phones with built in environmental sensors for air quality. There are several apps available, such as Plume, that display reported outdoor air quality and provide access to sensors for outdoor pollution, using official sensor grids. To monitor your indoor environment, you will need to purchase a hardware sensor device - most will measure several types of pollution in one device. You can assume a certain degree of protection if your dwelling is built to modern standards of ventilation but your own individual sensitivity to pollutants will determine if this is sufficient. Environmental actions arising may be as simple as opening a window, use of a humidifier/dehumidifier or better regulation of the temperature. You may also need to look at the choice of cleaning products or paints in use in your home if you need to create a purer environment.

Among the devices that can measure and report on your environment to your phone are:

- Withings Home - In perhaps a slightly surprising mixture of functionality, Withings - a pioneering company in personal health technology that produces several of the popular products mentioned in this book (Withings Body Analyzer Scales, Home Blood Pressure monitor, Aura Sleep system, Activite Step Counting watches and Pulse Ox Activity and HRM clip-on) - has decided to combine a VOC sensor into a High Definition Home Security camera, called the Home. This device which is about ¾ of the size of a soda can alerts you to movement in a room, as well as VOC levels. If they reach unhealthy levels the device blinks red and sends you a notification. With this data at hand you are able to make timely decisions, like opening the windows when using cleaning products.

- Air Mentor Pro - If you want to also track PM, then you need a more specialized device - something like the Air Mentor Pro which focuses exclusively on environmental matters. This triangular shaped device can either stand on a shelf or hang from a hook and measures temperature, humidity, VOC, $PM_{2.5}$ and PM_{10} - it can operate for up to 24 hours on its internal battery but is designed to be plugged in for normal operation. It both flashes a light and alerts its companion app if the air quality requires your attention. As a reference, it also provides local outdoor pollution information in the app, where it's available. It my case, its nearest information related to the other side of the city, about 5 miles from where I live, but probably reasonably indicative of my urban environment.

Skin & Sunshine

After all this talk about the quality and composition of the air in your house, you may be tempted to run outside for some sunshine and fresh air. And while I am of course an advocate of getting up and out for exercise, if you live somewhere sunny, there is the threat from sunshine if you do spend long periods outside or in intense sunshine.

While the talk of environmental pollutants so far has been largely centered on the associated respiratory health threats, another large public health issue in recent years has been exposure to sun, and the associated risk of skin cancer. Monitoring your sun exposure requires understanding of both UV-A and UV-B - the two types of UV radiation from the Sun that reach us through the Ozone layer (which absorbs most of the UV-B shorter wave-length rays). It is important to point out that sunlight has important positive physical effects when absorbed in moderation: UVB induces production of vitamin D in the skin and exposure to light is increasingly seen as important in positively influencing mood. Sunshine is essential as a natural source of vitamin D. It promotes bone health, prevents many chronic diseases and synchronizes the hormonal rhythms of our body.

Most people know that overexposure to sunlight can have damaging short term and long term impacts on skin. Yet, as with so many other health related topics, people are often slow to take action in the absence of a clear and present danger. From sunburn, to wrinkles and even skin cancer, our body's protective layer, which has an area of up to 2 square meters, can face quite an onslaught from the invisible power of the sun and its ultraviolet rays. There are 3.5 million cases of skin cancer in the United States each year, yet fewer than one third of people use sunscreen regularly, according to a report released by the Centers for Disease Control and Prevention.

A common refrain from people who don't actively protect their skin from sun exposure is that they didn't think they were getting enough exposure for it to be a problem. And in fairness, the variability of the sun's intensity can make managing your risk slightly tricky. It's also significant to note that different skin types respond differently to sun. The most common classification of Skin types is the Fitzpatrick Scale, developed by a Harvard dermatologist, which assigns one of six ratings based on reaction to UV light. This scale is frequently used in apps to offer skin-type specific guidance.

Sun exposure is yet another well-being related field where technology may offer convenient information and accessible, timely advice. There are already several technology-assisted solutions available that don't depend on mobiles or apps for their operation. Wrist bands like Sunfriend ($50) and stand-alone handheld monitors like SPC's UV Checker ($40) among others give you similar UVA and UVB tracking abilities at affordable prices without relying on your phone for trending, storage and alerting. But as has so frequently been the case throughout this book, the omnipresence of the mobile and the benefits it brings in terms of reminders, customizability of advice and trending of information over time make this yet another category that has seen dramatic growth in recent years.

Sun: App Solutions

Before we look at sensor-based solutions, let's look at the app-only offerings in this segment.

In their simplest form, apps in this category provide simple location-based UV index information such as the Environmental Protection Agency's free Sunwise UV Index app. This offers location or zip-code based hour-by-hour forecasts for UV index on a scale of 1 to 11+, where 11+ represents extreme risk of sunburn. Looking for the positives in sun exposure as a source of Vitamin D, the DMinder app is a Vitamin D tracking app. It uses GPS to determine your location and then computes when you can get vitamin D, how much of it you can make and gives you a timer. It also allows you to track Vitamin D intake from supplements and foods as well as your average weekly sun exposure levels.

The next stage of sophistication is to supplement this forecast information with individually relevant contextual information - one such app called SunZapp, developed in association with the National Cancer Institute combines GPS-based location information from the National Oceanic and Atmospheric Administration's UV Index forecast, with your personal information (skin tone, age, natural hair colour, eye colour and your clothes). This app also queries if you've taken any of a range of 20 common Over the Counter (OTC) medicines that increase your sensitivity from normal to sunlight and propensity to burn. Based on that information, it calculates how long it will take for you to suffer sunburn. A timer also highlights the time left until it is recommended that you reapply your sunscreen.

These apps all come with strong warnings that reliance on forecast information is not the same as reliance on actual locale-specific detected warnings. They also caution they are not medical-grade advisors.

Integrated Sensors

Samsung have included a UV sensor along with all the other health-related sensors mentioned earlier in their Note 4 and S6 phones, and updated the accompanying S-Health app to track UV levels. As with previous discussion on the benefits of integrated sensors, it is very convenient to have them always with you, requiring no additional pairing or charging but, by virtue of being built in, they are less discoverable (many owners may never realize they have it) and designed for ad-hoc readings rather than continuous monitoring. The Microsoft Band is currently unique among Fitness Trackers in including a UV sensor amongst its features.

Dedicated Devices

An example of a dedicated device to monitor sun and report it to an app via Bluetooth is the jewelry-styled wearable device called June from the same company that makes the Personal Weather station and indoor environment monitor mentioned earlier, Netatmo. It can be worn as a bracelet or a brooch and measures your sun exposure throughout the day, along with a daily sun forecast of UV index, as well as advice on whether you need sunscreen, sunglasses and/or a hat. It offers personalized advice based on a profile it creates from a one time questionnaire that asks about natural eye and hair color, skin tone, and how skin responds to sun without protection. Throughout the day, it will use live readings of UV via its sensor and update its advice regarding sunscreen application information or protective clothing and it will send you an alert when you're reaching the end of a safe amount of sun exposure.

A similar product to June in concept, though less female-targeted in its design, is the Violet. It's a small, waterproof clip-on tracker that gives real-time UV exposure information as well as notifications of potential skin damage. As an added feature, it also displays the daily natural vitamin D production based on actual sun exposure.

Using the aforementioned Fitzpatrick Scale, it classifies your skin and then calculates safe UV exposure time and required exposure time for recommended Vitamin D. You can also enter your clothing and sunscreen to get updated readings as well as setting a timer so the app reminds you when you've reached your limit with a notification.

SunSprite

The SunSprite clip-on sun monitor began life as a crowd-funded initiative. It measures the wearer's sunlight and UV exposure so as to ensure exposure to enough, but not too much, sunlight. Bluetooth connects it to a nearby smartphone but it provides on-device information via 10 LEDs which signify progress towards the recommended light exposure, with the lights flashing excitedly once you've reached 100%. The app provides historic information on both the light exposure (in LUX) and the UV levels. One outstanding feature of the SunSprite compared to any device mentioned in this entire volume is that it is completely solar-powered. So unlike every other device here, I've never had to plug it in to charge. For that reason alone, it's one of the easiest to use devices out there.

The SunSprite focuses on the positives of sunlight alongside the risks from over-exposure. The literature accompanying the app emphasizes the scientific studies over the last 30 years that point to light therapy as an effective treatment (vs medication) for depression as well as further research pointing to potential bright light benefits for a wide range of medical conditions including insomnia, ADHD, Parkinson's disease, and dementia.

Sun Education Remains a Challenge

While all of the sun protection devices and apps have potential, there remains the very real challenge of persuading people to use them. In January, JAMA Dermatology published mixed results on the effect of electronic reminders to use sunscreen. People who used an app used more sun protection techniques than those who didn't, but overall use of the tested app was lower than expected.

In June 2015 the Royal Pharmaceutical Society noted that there is huge confusion over the labels on sun creams, and urged that sun care manufacturers should all use the same rating system. A survey of 2,000 UK adults found one in five was unaware that the SPF rating does not mean protection against all sun damage - only that from UVB rays. UVA protection is measured on a separate "Star" rating on the packaging. This needs to improve urgently in the context that overexposure to ultraviolet radiation is the main preventable cause of skin cancers - both malignant melanoma and non-melanoma skin cancers, according to Cancer Research UK.

Cosmetics and Concerns

Aside from monitoring exposure to sunlight, careful consideration of and care for your skin is an important part of many people's well-being regime. Whether this is motivated by a skin complaint such as dermatitis, rashes and psoriasis, concern for melanoma or purely cosmetic considerations, there is a variety of devices, apps and services to cater for these issues.

Moles

Moles are the most common skin deformity and most people have between 30 and 40 moles, but some have as many as 600. A qualified dermatologist should be consulted to comprehensively evaluate moles, but there is a growing number of sources of information available to consumers keen to evaluate their own skin either before or as a trigger for a professional consultation. Both the American Association of Dermatologists and the National Cancer Institute provide extensive guidelines for consumers urging them to check themselves for potential abnormalities. As a guide, the mnemonic ABCDE is used - Asymmetry, Border, Color, Diameter and Evolution.

Doctors and dermatologists typically use a device called a dermatoscope to assess moles and while the price of these devices has dropped considerably to an almost-consumer level of about $700, there is not yet a widely available and truly affordable consumer device. And in the absence of such a solution, app developers have once again stepped in.

The emergence of cameras as ubiquitous on modern phones has led to the creation of numerous photo-sharing services of remarkable popularity such as Instagram and Flickr. More photographs are now taken daily with phones than with cameras, and while the majority of them are for leisure purposes, there is a growing number of specialist apps that take advantage of the ability to capture and send photos nearly instantly. We'll look at one aimed at doctors called Figure One in a later chapter but for now, I want to focus on apps that are designed to help identify worrying skin conditions.

There are several popular apps for mole checking that enable you to submit photos of moles for "professional" evaluation. Apps can give you a useful record of a mole over time to help identify any changes (which is a key indicator of a potential problem) as well as providing a convenient reminder to check a mole, which may not be easily remembered but it is vital to point out that relying on an app of unknown origin/medical expertise for diagnostic purposes is foolhardy at best and irresponsible at worst. As we'll discuss in the chapter on regulation, there have already been examples of apps in this sphere purporting to offer capabilities that have met with strong disapproval from the FDA. Personally, I'm in favor of using reputable apps as a first step in monitoring your skin, but with the strong provision that if you are in any doubt based on ABCDE, you should urgently consult a professional, even if the app says it's ok. You don't want to become one of the 10,000 people who die from skin cancer in the US alone each year!

Routine Skin Analysis

While protecting yourself from overexposure as well as seeking advice in the event of any changes in your skin are important, many people may be interested in additional advice, tailored to their skin, in order to optimize their cosmetic and skin-care expenditure.

- An example of a device that both monitors external skin influences such as UV and humidity levels as well as enabling detailed analysis of your skin itself is called the Wave. Clearly designed to appeal aesthetically to females, this comes in a device the size and style of a make-up compact. Wave uses bio electrical impedance to analyzes the moisture content & oil balance of your skin and displays this trended on your app, along with recommendations as to what action to take in the event of for example dehydration, which would require moisturization. Simply touch the device to your skin for 3 seconds and it will report on the moisture and oil content of your skin at that point.

- Another example of a consumer-oriented device originating from professional/clinical environments is the OKU. This small cube-shaped scanner enables consumers to see below their skin's surface and analyze and address their skincare concerns. Using dermography and spectroscopy to analyze your skin, the device analyzes this information and gives a detailed assessment of the skin in a measurement called a skin score, made up of details on moisture, texture, oil, wrinkles, and pigmentation. At $299 and recommended for use twice a day, this is going to appeal to people who are particularly interested in their skin's well-being more than to the casual observer, but as with all the technologies here, its value is very much relative to the benefit each user sees in its results.

Several of the sun-monitoring apps and devices advise you on when you need sunglasses to protect your eyes and that is the next area we're going to look at where mobile technology is making an impact.

Optical Health

Of all of the medical disciplines, it is perhaps ophthalmology more than most that has already seen obvious technology-led change in recent years. Advances in imaging technology mean that photographs of the inside of your eye are now a standard element of a high-street eye test, and manufacturing and materials advances means we can expect custom prescriptions to be available in an hour.

If you want an accessory to turn your iPhone into a fully-fledged Ophthalmoscope that lets you see and photograph the fundus (interior surface of the eye opposite the lens) of the eye, you can do so at a cost of approx $600 but of course most people wouldn't have any idea what to look for! Eye care is a complex field and while I strongly advise people to seek professional medical care, when it comes to looking after your eyes, you may need to see an Ophthalmologist, an Orthoptist, an Optometrist or an Optician or some combination of them all! Such complexity provides a warning that you shouldn't expect too much from your phone but there are still ways that it can help you to learn more about these precious organs.

Popular free app Eyecare plus offers a fairly bewildering array of tests to work your way through. While perhaps quicker and more convenient to try on your smartphone, it does take some time to complete the tests. Some are exercises you must complete while others are questions you must answer. And since it says to hold at arm's length for many of the tests, this may be an occasion you'll be glad you opted for a large screen phone ;)

- Visual acuity - acuteness and clearness of vision by showing you a succession of smaller and smaller images as you hold your phone at arm's length

- Accommodation - level of vision accommodation at different distances by asking you a series of questions about the frequency you encounter conditions likes red eyes or blurred visions or headaches.

- Cataract test - series of questions

- Contrast Sensitivity - similar to visual acuity, shows you a series of images at arm's length but varies their color/contrast with the background

- Red Desaturation - shows you a red background and then a small red image and you have to judge if they were the same share of red

- Central vision - shows you a grid and checks if you observed any waviness of lines

- Color blindness - reveals RGB weaknesses by showing you numbers or patterns hidden in combinations of colors and by asking you to arrange a series of color blocks in saturation order.

It also includes the ability to submit a question to a doctor along with advice on healthy food and eye care tips. In order to encourage you to return and complete the tests frequently, the app uses a points system to motivate you to repeat tests and underlying this gamification is the fact that as with many indicators mentioned in this book, changes in results are a clear sign to seek professional interpretation. Alongside the tests, the app also provides trainings, exercises to improve your vision and prevent issues. These on-screen patterns and motions are designed to give your eyes a work-out as well as train the muscles and focus.

Assistance for Visually Impaired

Pharmaceutical giant Novartis has released a series of apps for the visually impaired as well as an app for doctors to help explain vision issues to patients.

ViaOpta Daily and Nav are two apps that offer people with visual impairment apps designed to be easier to use, with larger buttons, various contrast modes and voice guides. The Daily app includes a feature that uses the phone's camera to audibly identify money denominations (Euro and Dollars) as well as colours. The Nav app is intended to help visually impaired users to find locations more easily.

ViaOpta simulator allows a doctor to show the effect of different eye conditions on vision by showing the impact using the phone or tablet camera. It alters the camera feed to illustrate how each condition manifests itself. The user can alter the severity of the effect in the app. Although targeted at healthcare professionals, patients can download and use the app to better understand eye conditions. The current version covers the following conditions:

- Wet age-related macular degeneration
- Dry age-related macular degeneration
- Myopic choroidal neovascularization
- Diabetic retinopathy
- Diabetic macular edema
- Central retinal vein occlusion
- Branch retinal vein occlusion
- Glaucoma
- Cataract
- Vitreomacular traction/macular hole

Promise for the Developing World

While eye test and exercise apps may offer benefits in between visits to your optician or prompt you to visit one if you notice something amiss, mobile technology may offer the greatest benefits for eye health in the developing world where problems are more common and access to opticians far less readily available - of the 285 million people in the world with vision impairment, 80 percent live in low-income countries. The vast majority have preventable or treatable conditions, like glaucoma or cataracts. A study recently published in the journal JAMA Ophthalmology, demonstrated that a smartphone based vision test was as accurate as the other two methods for testing vision. However, even if inexpensive smartphone-based tests can extend eye examinations to developing countries, the associated potential to save eyesight can only be realized if the required treatments are made as available as the diagnostic advances.

Are you Sitting Comfortably?

Then I'll begin! While the earlier chapter on the importance of tracking your activity may have frightened you into never sitting still again, it is of course impractical for most people, with many of us spending large portions of our day sat in front of a desk or screen or steering wheel. One of the most immediately noticeable features of the Apple Watch is the insistent tap on your wrist it delivers if you've been sat still for 50 minutes, admonishing you to stand up and walk around for a minute every hour. And even if you do manage to take on board the advice to get up and move around frequently, you will likely still spend several hours a day sitting still.

The act of sitting now also has a choice of sensors to make sure you're "doing it right". Most of us don't remember learning how to sit, but some people sit better than others - maintaining a better posture. Back pain is a very real problem - just ask anyone who suffers from it. In fact, it is the second most common reason for missing work and visits to the doctor in the US. Minimizing the risk of back trouble begins with maintaining good posture. It's not something most people think about, and many of us have bad habits when it comes to how we prefer to sit.

While back pain may be the most obvious outcome of bad sitting habits, a lack of attention to your sitting habits may also increase your risk for neck pain, varicose veins and joint pains. With the average daily time spent sitting now over 9 hours compared to only 7 hours a generation ago, significant amounts of research into the impacts of sitting on our well-being have been conducted. They make for some frightening reading and reinforce the importance of regular activity we discussed earlier. And when you're required by your job to sit for extended periods of time, it's worth considering the quality of how you sit so as to minimize the negative impacts on your body. If you'd like some more statistics on the dangers of sitting, check out this infographic: http://visual.ly/sitting-killing-you

While activity trackers, smart watches and some phones can be set to remind you if you've been inactive for long, these types of generic solutions don't focus on how you are being inactive. They don't differentiate between you sitting still but bolt upright and a lack of movement when you are slumped or hunched over a desk.

The more extreme solutions to too much sitting include stand-up desks and treadmill desks. These are pretty expensive and not practical in many work situations but luckily I've come across two mobile-centric solutions to help people suffering from posture problems. The simplest is the Lumo Lift - a small device that clips magnetically to your clothes near your collarbone. It then monitors your posture and vibrates gently if your posture slips from the desired angle for too long. A more insistent coaching mode is also provided that vibrates as soon as your posture slips from the ideal, rather than giving you time to recover like the alert mode. The little device simultaneously reports your steps to the app (and onwards to a calorie tracking app such as MyFitness Pal if desired) as well as providing graphs showing the trends of your posture, over months or days, right down to the hour. This may help you identify if there are particular times of the day or particular locations that are more associated with bad posture.

The posture-promoting products from Lumo are a good example of the rapid progress these kinds of devices make. The first generation product (called Lumo Back) was a relatively large black device that you had to strap on at the base of your back using a belt. The second generation device is much more user-friendly small clip for your collarbone area, that is even available in a fashionable range of colors and even embellished with crystals. This little device clips on to your shirt near your collarbone and once calibrated (by a simple double push of the button while you're standing upright), it will remind you with a vibration throughout the day if you start to slump. The app displays how many hours of the day you managed to maintain a good posture.

Approaching the issue of posture from a completely different perspective is the Darma - the world's first smart cushion. I have to admit I did a double-take the first time I heard of this product, but when you think about it, monitoring sitting from the perspective of the chair may have its merits. Obviously less portable than the wearable solution discussed above, Darma is aimed at those people who spend a lot of time sitting in one place. But this approach allows it to measure more than just the angle you're sitting at.

Although not strictly a wearable technology, Darma Smart cushion ($200) shares many features with this trendy category of hardware given its health emphasis and reliance on a mobile phone for display and processing power. It has the added benefit of not being something you need to remember to wear, and once in place on your seat (most likely at work), you can leave it there. Needing to be charged once a month, the cushion uses Ballistocardiography (BCG) technology to track your heart rate with medical accuracy.

The Darma Smart Cushion uses an accompanying app to illustrate if you're sitting correctly based on the pressure you're exerting on the cushion's sensors, providing you real time feedback and it teaches you to sit properly, by extending the spine and engaging your core muscles. It also prompts you to move to a standing position when you're overdue a position change, and all the while you're sitting on it, the device is measuring your heartbeat and respiration rate which are key indicators of stress.

Oral Health

Even your mouth hasn't escaped the onslaught of technology. Despite the fact that my dentist has for years used text messages to remind me I'm overdue for my next check-up, I hadn't thought about technology being of benefit to my oral health, and in fact had forgotten that one of the most prevalent mobile technologies, Bluetooth has quite a big hint in the name! Although I don't believe for a second that the Ericsson engineers who named the low-power, short-range wireless communication technology after Viking Harald Bluetooth ever really envisaged their technology ending up in an actual toothbrush as the term "Bluetooth toothbrush" is a bit of a mouthful. Pun intended.

Given the gravity of some of the topics already covered in this book, avoiding cavities may sound like a fairly low priority - should you really care about your oral health? Well if you realize that your oral health can offer clues about your overall health — or that problems in your mouth can affect the rest of your body, you might want to pay slightly more attention to it as not only a means to avoid unpleasant trips to the dreaded dentist.

Taking good care of your mouth, teeth and gums is a worthy goal in and of itself. Good oral and dental hygiene can help prevent bad breath, tooth decay and gum disease—and can help you keep your teeth as you get older. An unhealthy mouth, especially if you have gum disease, may increase your risk of serious health problems such as heart attack, stroke, and even poorly controlled diabetes.

Bluetooth Toothbrush

Electric toothbrushes have been around for a long time, so the concept of charging your toothbrush is already well established. What is new is the advent of smart toothbrushes, that pack sensors and wireless communications into the slightly chubbier than average handle.

The apps that accompany these next-generation oral cleaning devices offer reminders to brush, diagrams of where to brush, as well as logging the exact time spent in each quadrant of your mouth. When you've finished brushing, they may also recommend additional cleansing in the form of mouthwash or flossing. Models are available from established players like Oral-B and startups such as Kolibree.

Breathometer

Beyond routine and effective brushing support, mobile technology is now available to assess your breath quality. Gone are the days of blowing into your hand and trying to smell if a breath freshener was required. Enter the Breathometer Mint - a handheld device you simply blow into for a scientific assessment of any nasty smells emanating from your mouth that might cause you social problems, or worse still be a symptom of impending oral health issues.

The science behind breath quality involves Volatile Sulfur Compounds (VSCs), not to be confused with the VOCs from earlier, as these are created by bacteria in the mouth. Elevated levels may indicate gum disease and tooth decay but are associated with reduced breath quality. For anyone looking for more scientific detail, the associated website proudly proclaims that their device measures: Hydrogen Sulfide, Methyl Mercapthan and Hydrogen Disulfide levels in parts per billion. I bet you never even knew you had them in your mouth!

Hydration

We touched on hydration earlier in the vital signs section and mentioned it above when talking about skin, but it's worth highlighting again here the importance of drinking adequate water. Whether you're a serious athlete, leisurely exerciser, or just trying to stay healthy, it's important to make sure you drink the right amount of water before, during and after exercising. If you're not properly hydrated, your body will be unable to perform at its highest level, and you may experience fatigue, muscle cramps, dizziness or more serious symptoms.

Surveys show that most people are actually frequently slightly dehydrated despite thinking they drink quite a lot - relying on other fluids besides water. The bad news is that coffee, tea, alcohol and sodas don't count the same as pure water; they're diuretics, which means they actually remove water and nutrients from the body.

Along with checking your breath quality, the Breathometer Mint device also provides information about the state of oral hydration and allows you to track hydration level trends. Of course if you do need to take action to track your hydration levels, you may need to consider a smart water bottle. Yes, I did say smart water bottle - surely you're not surprised by now that such a thing exists?

Smart waters bottles aren't a brand new concept. A few years ago, I did have a water bottle that tracked consumption and displayed how many litres I had consumed on a small LCD screen on the front of the bottle. However, because it wasn't linked to anything that actually recorded what I was drinking, I quickly ignored it. I'm fairly sure I'll pay much closer attention to my forthcoming bluetooth enabled one that will deliver my hydration compliance straight to my phone.

The HidrateMe (sic) is a $40 smart water bottle that holds 24oz of water with a sensor stick inside the bottle that automatically tracks how much you drink throughout the day. It sends information to the app on your phone to track consumption over time and the bottle glows when it's time to drink more water just in case a reminder on your phone isn't enough motivation.

Did You Hear?

Lest we leave any orifice untouched by technology, let's finally for this chapter turn our attention to the ears. Perhaps often the innocent victim of loud music via the increased amounts of music provided by phones (According to the World Health Organization, some 1.1 billion teenagers and young adults are at risk of hearing loss due to the unsafe use of personal audio devices, including smartphones, and exposure to damaging levels of sound at noisy entertainment venues such as nightclubs, bars and sporting events), it is good to know that phones have been adapted to help rather than bombard our ears.

Worldwide it is estimated that up to 360 million people have moderate to profound hearing loss due to various causes, such as noise, genetic conditions, complications at birth, certain infectious diseases, chronic ear infections, the use of particular drugs, and ageing. It is believed as many as 50% of all cases of hearing loss are avoidable. Transient Hearing difficulties may also be as simple as an ear infection or the build-up of wax. Safe exposure to noise depends on the intensity or loudness of sound, and the duration and frequency of listening. Exposure to loud sounds can result in temporary hearing loss or tinnitus which is a ringing sensation in the ear. When the exposure is particularly loud, regular or prolonged, it can lead to permanent damage of the ear's sensory cells, resulting in irreversible hearing loss. WHO recommends that the highest permissible level of noise exposure in the workplace is 85 dB up to a maximum of eight hours per day. Noise can also be considered an environmental pollutant and is measured by some of the environmental and sleep sensors mentioned earlier.

Sound Meter

Most phones now include warnings if you try to turn the volume up to dangerous levels when playing music. "Loud" noises such as those in some workplaces or entertainment venues are harder to quantify without a sound meter. Yet again, we see the mobile phone and app developers stepping in to create approximate but accessible alternatives to previously exclusively professional measuring solutions. For example, the Swedish Government Work Environment Authority has published a Noise Meter app, with the caution that "The application is not the equivalent of a professional noise calculator, but it gives approximate values." It offers both a decibel meter that measures the sound level in real time and a noise calculator where you can work out how much noise you are exposed to during an 8-hour day. Intended to assist workers who may be exposed to severe workplace noise levels to quickly assess if a more professional review is required, it boasts over 100,000 downloads. It quotes Swedish noise regulations which state that employers are required to inform employees of the risks associated with levels of 80dB and above, as well as requiring them to provide hearing protection.

Hearing Test

Not to be out done by eye tests, there are also apps available for hearing tests. The eponymously named Hearing Test app uses headphones with your phone to determine the quietest audible sound in both the left and right ears. It plays a pure audio tone at a variety of frequencies which you then indicate when you can no longer hear it. A graph shows your relative performance and can indicate if you suffer from mild to severe hearing loss.

Examining the ears

An otoscope (or auriscope) is the medical device used to look into the ear during examinations outside of specialist ENT facilities where more sophisticated devices may be available. Domestic otoscopes are available (from as little as £5) and may be of particular interest to people who suffer from recurring ear infections. However, while a parent may use a domestic otoscope to establish if a child has an ear infection, they are unlikely to be able to interpret what they see. A start-up in California has tackled this using mobile technology. Cellscope has created an attachment for an iPhone that enables you to record a video of the inside of the ear and then either show it to your physician or send it directly to an online service which (at a cost of $49) will provide a written diagnosis and treatment plan within 2 hours, 24x7.

Vitamins & Minerals

The human body requires a variety of vitamins and minerals in varying quantities to function properly. Vitamins are organic substances, while Minerals are inorganic substances. The body cannot produce them itself and so they must be obtained through diet. There is a recommended daily allowance for each type of nutrient that you should get by eating specific food types naturally rich in certain vitamins or minerals, or that have been fortified with compounds you might otherwise struggle to ingest in sufficient quantities.

In 2013, the global market for vitamins and supplements exceeded $90 billion, growing at a compound annual growth rate (CAGR) of 5% according to Euromonitor. Vitamins and minerals pills dominate the shelves of many supermarkets, health shops and pharmacies - but unless you are sure you actually need them, what you are doing is creating expensive urine as the body is not always able to store these substances (especially Vitamins A, B, E, and K) and needs a constant supply of them through a balanced diet. Exceeding the daily amount for a particular vitamin or mineral may be harmful, but should you be deficient in one or more of them, knowing that and knowing what to take to alleviate it may have very positive benefits.

You may be wondering, beyond offering dietary advice, how your mobile phone could help with understanding vitamins and minerals, but once again, technology has seized on the opportunity provided by the processing power and display possibilities afforded by phones and paired your phone with a miniaturized version of sensor technology (EAV) that was previously the size of a small suitcase in a clinical setting. Most people who have vitamin or mineral deficiencies or imbalances are not aware of these until the associated symptoms manifest themselves. With domestic testing, it is possible to identify these issues before the harms they cause become apparent.

The Vitastiq is shaped like a large pen and connects to your phone by a wire (no bluetooth connection here to save cost and remove the need for a rechargeable battery). You then press it against various points on your body as directed in the app and as you move it across each of your fingers and toes and a few other select body areas, you can watch as it measures some 30 different vitamins and minerals:

Bile Acid	Magnesium	Vitamin B12
Biotin	Manganese	Vitamin B2
Calcium	Omega 3-6 fatty	Vitamin B3
Chromium	acids	Vitamin B5
Coenzyme Q10	Pepsin	Vitamin B6
Copper	Potassium	Vitamin C
Folic Acid (B9)	Proteins	Vitamin D
Glucosamine	Selenium	Vitamin E
Haemoglobin	Sodium	Zinc
Iodine	Vitamin A	
Iron	Vitamin B1	

Thankfully, the app includes a detailed description of each substance measured, as well as advice on what foods contain sources of it, and the possible implications of abnormal levels. The device uses Electro-Acupuncture (EAV) to measure the electrical conductance at body areas based on Chinese acupuncture traditions. This is totally non-invasive yet offers a lot of insight into the internal composition of your body.

The Importance of Medicines

So far we've dealt primarily with the explosion of devices and software that are intended to help with diagnosis or monitoring of symptoms. Whether or not the diagnosis of a condition originates from a mobile-assisted point of view, some form of medication is the most common outcome of a visit to a physician. In 2010, 2.6 billion drugs were ordered or provided by US Physicians, excluding hospitals. In any given month, virtually half (48.7% according to the CDC) of the entire US population take a prescription medicine, while one in 10 take more than 5 drugs.

In the words of Paracelsus the renowned 16th century Swiss German physician, botanist and alchemist: "The dosage makes it either a poison or a remedy." Nonadherence (which applies to under as well as overdoses) to prescribed dosing regimens can have severe negative effects on patient health. It's also hugely expensive, leading to an estimated $100 billion in additional or avoidable annual healthcare costs, according to research published in the August 4, 2005, New England Journal of Medicine. When long-term medication is prescribed, fully half of patients fail to adhere to the prescribed regimen, European research has found. The increase in so-called polypharmacy (the taking of more than 4 prescription medications at once) has led to some patients being under a dauntingly complex, several times daily pill burden.

Compliance or Adherence is not just a simple matter of people forgetting to take their medicine which can be fixed with a reminder. While that can of course be the case, much research points to evidence of people choosing not to take their prescribed medicine or dosage. This can be for a variety of reasons such as: side effects, lack of belief in the drugs, the costs or impatience with a lack of immediate results - especially common for cholesterol or blood pressure drugs where the patient is asymptomatic and may remain so for many years without the drugs.

In cases where it is side effects that persuade a person to stop taking pills, capturing this is valuable research data. Dr Ben Goldacre makes this point very strongly in his book Bad Pharma that those who drop out of trials due to side effects are a significant factor in reducing the quality of clinical trials and clinical trials data. The NHS in the UK operate a web site - yellowcard.mhra.gov.uk that enables patients and health professionals alike to report side effects, defective/poor quality medicine, fake medicine or adverse incidents with medical devices. If you find yourself encountering issues with medicine or medical devices, then you should report it.

A Pill For Every Ill And There's An App For That...

If technologists are sometimes overly keen to answer any issue by pointing out that there's an app for that, doctors and pharmaceutical companies have been accused in the past of answering every ill with "there's a pill for that". So it was probably inevitable that the two would meet - there's now a plethora of apps about pills.

For inadvertent non-adherence to pill taking regimens, there are of course already plenty of non-technical solutions - speaking alarm clocks as well as all manner of digital and mechanical pill boxes with intricate chambers for each dose. But as is the recurring theme of this book, existing solutions can be enhanced with the kind of reminders, tracking and communication features made possible by mobile technologies.

Although it's yet to be measured, medical adherence may increase based on the uptake of several of the technologies referred to earlier - a kind of positive side effect all too often missing from medical discussions! Constant heart rate measurement and simple home blood pressure monitoring, for example, may make people more aware of their heart health and more open to taking constant doses of tablets despite any apparent symptoms, as the readings may suffice as motivators.

Once again, the technology breaks down into app-only solutions and appcessories where apps support dedicated hardware that tries to tackle the problem. There is little research yet as to the efficacy of these solutions - a 2013 article in the Journal of the American Pharmacists Association noted over 160 Smartphone Medication Adherence Apps but could only refer to potential benefits rather than demonstrable improvements - but this is a fast-moving area that will likely see rapid innovation in the coming years.

Medication Management Apps

There are numerous apps to remind you when to take your pills once you set them up with the prescribed dosage. Most include additional information above and beyond simple timed reminders to include recommendations about whether/when medicine should be taken in relation to meals. The more intelligent apps also offer visual guides to pills or even the ability to look up pill information based on shape, color and markings - helpful for people who may have multiple pills to take and risk cross-contamination.

- MyMeds.com offers a web and app-based adherence service for $10 a year that enables users to setup their own and their familie's medication records and store them securely on a cloud service.

- One of the most popular free apps in this space, Medisafe, boasts well over a million downloads. It extends beyond simple reminders by adding a social element with notifications and missed medications shared with your specified family members or caregiver. It will track your pill supply so as to remind you when you need to refill and you can choose to send a summary of your pill-taking to your doctor, assuming you have your doctor's email address.

For those wishing to fool compliance systems, most stop nagging you once you open the appointed container and trust you when you press the "I've taken it button". Ultimately, it is the patient who stands to suffer most from non-adherence, but it is not inconceivable that skin or blood tests via wearable devices or home testing kits may be required by those funding pills to verify actual compliance. At least in situations where adherence apps or devices are used, Doctors can know that non-compliance is willful on the part of the patient rather than accidental.

As a sector more commercially-minded than some others of the healthcare system, dispensing pharmacies have been relatively quick to roll out extensive app-based solutions to ensure a steady flow of prescription refills. Both Walgreens and CVS, as the two titans of the US drugstore landscape, offer apps to remind you to take your medications, manage your refills (even for family members with their consent) and scanners that enable you to reorder medicines with a simple barcode scan using your smartphone.

As we wrap up the summary of the technologies available and start to move on in the next chapter to the impacts of these and the policy decisions that may await us, it's timely to consider what impact seemingly simple technologies related to adherence may eventually have. As the pressures on health budgets grow, this area could attract a lot of attention and adherence tracking could become a requirement for patients taking drugs that are paid for by insurers. More of that in the next Chapter.

Head to Toe

So it seems like we have covered scanners and sensors for every conceivable part of the body. In researching this book, it is perhaps only the toes that have escaped the application of sensors and before you ask, there are plenty of hats that come with sensors so I think it's fair to say that you could be covered from head to toe in the years ahead. I thought toes had escaped but then I read about the smart insole and smart socks available!

There are many, many more specialized devices that it's just not practical to cover here. That is not to in any way minimize the importance to those affected by any ailment not covered in these pages. If you are suffering from a chronic condition, I urge you to investigate the apps and devices available that may be of benefit to you. There are apps to for hemophilia patients (Pfizer's HemMobile), Bluetooth Spirometers for Chronic Obstructive Pulmonary Disorder (COPD) sufferers and Bluetooth enabled inhalers for Asthmatics (Propeller Health) to name just a few more areas where care that was previously only available in clinics is now moving closer to patients and even into their homes. Where to start looking for developments in your particular field of interest? Check out the patient-centric sites in the next chapter.

Do I need it?

You may be left wondering which, if any, of the aforementioned apps and devices you may need. Remember that I am not trying to sell you any of these solutions. My perspective is that it's important to know what tools are available so you can make an informed decision if any of them could be of benefit to your very individual needs. It would be a tragedy to find yourself looking back from a hospital bed in years to come only learning then of an app or device that could have prevented you ending up there.

For devices, apps and services where there is perhaps a less obvious benefit (most people accept that activity is a good thing and don't seek reassurance while not as many people would be aware of the benefits of good posture), several of the innovators go to great lengths to convince potential customers of the science backing up their claims. On most web sites from the purveyors of these gadgets, you'll find endorsements from highly qualified medical professionals to lend credibility to the solution. My advice would be to research the solutions available that tackle areas of your well-being that you are concerned about, consult both online forums and your healthcare professional and then make your decision on whether a particular solution merits your time and money to try.

Chapter 9:
The Social Side of Medicine

"Top question of the dying: "What made me sick?"

- Steven Magee

The Scale of Sickness

There are of course very different levels of being sick. From a viral cold to a bacterial infection to any number of terminal or chronic illnesses, the WHO distinguishes 12,420 diseases in their latest ICD database, the international standard for classifying diseases. Contracting or discovering you have a disease can have significant psychological impacts alongside the more visible physiological outcomes. It can be as important to recognize this as to treat the physical disease. I won't distinguish in this chapter between types of disease (genetic, communicable, non-communicable, etc) or delve into the pedantic differences between illness, disease and disorder as terms - at this level, I include all medical conditions, real or perceived by patients.

If you've reflected on some of your lifestyle choices and the potential benefits that you might enjoy if you choose to improve them, you will find support in this chapter as we look at how technology can help motivate us to achieving a healthier lifestyle, alone or with the involvement of others. Then we'll examine how it can help us in better understanding conditions if and when they do develop when the social element switches from prevention to support. The final section of this chapter then looks beyond our own individual interest to see how mobile technology can be applied to helping others.

Motivation - Choosing And Keeping The Healthier Lifestyle

"We spend the first half of our lives making ourselves sick, and the second half of our lives trying to make ourselves un-sick."

– Kevin W. Reese

If we were completely rational creatures, more of us would prioritize adjusting our lifestyle in line with the best practices supported by evidence-based medicine in order to maximize our chances of leading a longer, healthier life. While much doubt exists in medicine, there are plenty of areas where clear proof exists of causal links between behaviors and adverse medical outcomes. Yet for a variety of reasons, many people choose not to adopt healthier lifestyles.

Still, there are large numbers of people who try to adopt healthier lifestyles and are willing to invest money into it - just see the spike in home fitness sales each Christmas - but the number of expensive treadmills and exercise bikes that are attracting dust by March is testimony to the difficulty in maintaining usage beyond the initial rush of enthusiasm. And it's here that phones play such a vital role - they can continue to advise you simply because they are always with you - and not relegated to the corner of the spare room with the rowing machine, hidden under a sheet….

Make it Fun, Scary or Just Economic

Mobile phones began their life as basic, if amazing, communication tools - enabling us to talk and text with people from anywhere. As they gained data functionality, they added email and now apps. Among the most popular apps remain communication apps where the sharing of text (What's App) and photos (Instagram) have in many cases come to supplant traditional voice and text as the dominant use of the smartphone. But a key trend in the socialization of mobiles has been the inclusion of social features in apps whose core purpose is not direct communication.

Virtually all the leading health apps offer the ability to share or to join a community. Even those that don't share, offer you contextual information about how your performance may compare to other users in similar age groups, locations or behavior cohorts as yours. One common trend among well-being/fitness apps regardless of whether they are trying to change your exercise, posture or diet, is their adoption of motivational social and so-called gamification features. Not that health is a game, but the concept of gamification is a key feature of many of the leading fitness and well-being apps. Based on the premise that people respond well to competitive challenges, progressive goals and acknowledgement of achievement, it is common to see leaderboards, friend invites and challenges in apps that began life as simple electronic diaries of record.

One Marshmallow or Two?

If self-control is something you believe you lack and cannot develop, there is great encouragement to be gleaned from the work of the Stanford psychologist Walter Mischel, who ran the so-called Marshmallow experiments in the late 1960s and early 1970s that examined delayed gratification. In the experiment, children were offered the choice between taking one marshmallow immediately, or two if they waited 15 minutes. Those children who were able to wait longer for the bigger rewards tended to have better life outcomes, as measured by college admission tests and BMI. The study, and many subsequent pieces, of research looked at the techniques children used to occupy themselves to wait more effectively for the larger but delayed rewards. These techniques such as visualization and distraction can be taught and developed.

With invisible health threats such as High Blood Pressure (Hypertension), and a frequent narcissistic instinct towards living for the moment, maintaining motivation towards a healthier lifestyle can be very challenging - even more so than resisting eating a marshmallow! As we'll see in a later chapter, there may be external factors that come to bear in the near future that will focus people more, but until then, let's look at the techniques employed by mobile apps to help us stay on the straight and narrow.

Shame or Reward

The simplest technique employed, but one with widespread appeal, is that of the "Streak". Put simply, the app counts the number of consecutive days you achieve your goal and reminds you if you're about to break your streak, with a silent implication that breaking it would be a very bad thing. "You've logged in for 220 days in a row - make sure you log in before Midnight to keep your streak going!" it prompts with a degree of urgency as it turns 8pm.

If the shame of breaking your streak is insufficient motivation, many apps are now trying a more rewarding approach, bestowing virtual badges as you pass particular milestones. "Congratulations on Unlocking the Concorde Badge - you've completed a lifetime elevation of 18,000 meters, the cruising altitude of the Concorde". How nice of them. "Still 2306 m before your next badge". Ah right, clearly I can't stop now without knowing what badge I'll win next?

And the Winner is...

For the competitive animal in all of us, the use of leaderboards may prove motivational - how do you steps compared so far this week against your mates? Or have you had that many more calories than your sibling? While the bragging rights of topping the leaderboard may work for some, others will be motivated to know how they compare to "people like you". Already a familiar concept from sites like Amazon, the curiosity to know how we compare and conform is strong. "People your age tend to sleep an average of 6h 42m each night, but you sleep for 5h 54m" or "Your 132,000 steps last week places you in the top 3% of users worldwide".

Matchup allows you to create and participate in activity challenges with friends or groups of other Matchup users. Working with multiple different trackers so you don't all have to have the same device, this app allows you create your own competition, set a prize, and challenge your friends or colleagues. If you're looking for additional motivation, the service offers ready-made challenges such as sustain an average of 25,000 steps for 7 days.

Taking the concept of gamification literally, the Atari Fit app offers over 100 gamified exercise routines including full-body circuits and running programs, designed and certified in association with the National Academy of Sports Medicine. Users can unlock additional fitness routines with points earned from burning calories (or through in-app purchases). Users can also import their data from wearable devices or other services to earn in-game rewards. If you raise your fitness level in Atari Fit you receive virtual coins which unlock access to classic Atari titles such as Pong and Super Breakout. A tie-up with Walgreens means you can also unlock discounts at the US pharmacy stores.

Make It Pay

And If virtual badges and the social honor of topping a leaderboard or being in the top cohort worldwide aren't enough to energize you to get some exercise, what about cold hard cash? Pact is an app that lets you win money for sticking to your exercise goals, but costs you money if you don't. So once you've downloaded Pact and setup an account, you are asked to set your goal. For example, you commit to logging your caloric intake 6 days a week. If you do it tells you, you'll earn about $1. So far so good, if not exactly a life-changing payout to anticipate. Then you have to set your forfeit - you have to enter the stake you'll pay if you don't hit your 6 day logging goal - the stake you'll pay each and every single day you miss. It starts with a recommendation of $10. Next step enter your credit card or PayPal account. Gulp!! For the unsure among you, there is an option to try it without the monetary rewards or penalties if you want to see how it goes, but where's the fun in that? Most behavior modification study shows that habits formed based on rewards are sustainable so if you can find the right reward, you will increase your chances of long-term success.

Scare Tactics - Zombies or Espionage!

Still not convinced these techniques will keep you motivated? What about fear then? In this case I don't mean fear of dying young or suffering a slow and painful illness, I mean death at the hands of flesh-eating zombies? Is that enough to make you walk a bit faster? Apparently one app developer thinks it just might be and has created a popular app that tries this bit of escapism. I could have mentioned these under activity tracking earlier but they more properly seem to me to belong here under the heading of motivational tools.

Zombies, Run! is an immersive running game and audio adventure that has attracted over 1,000,000 users. Each workout you embark upon becomes a mission where you're the hero at the center of your very own zombie adventure story. The App works at any speed though it may seem like cheating to merely walk when you've zombies to evade! You get a certain number of "missions" for free or pay $20 a year for access to all the stories. If you are running the story unfolds in between tracks you add to a playlist, through a series of dynamic radio messages and voice recordings.

A less terrifying variant of the concept has been commissioned from the same app company by the NHS in the UK, which replaces the Zombies with espionage-style storytelling. Simply called "The Walk", the plot requires you to solve a bombing where you're rewarded for walking more by collecting clues, scanning for information, and unlocking achievements. It is adaptive, meaning it adjusts its difficulty based on individual fitness levels. To stay alive, you'll need to walk the length of the UK. and the NHS is hoping you're motivated to actually get your exercise so you can progress further into the story while evading capture by the police and enemy agents.

Do Buddies Really Help?

The app makers claim that those who buddy up for exercise perform dramatically better. For example, Jawbone data shows that users of their UP app who have three or more friends on their team move 10 extra miles a month and Fitbit claim that their users with one or more friends are 27% more active. I'd like to see an independent systematic review of these kinds of claims but until we have one of them, I have no reason to believe that the app companies aren't being truthful. However, when assessing claims, you do need to be watchful for funding bias or cherry-picking of results!

Each app typically provides its own closed community to avoid over-sharing on Facebook, though most offer the chance to find friends via the established social networks. Even if you are "pumped" about your new found motivation and interest in activity, consider before you share every step you take - your social circle may be happy for your health, but may be decidedly unhappy if you feel the need to update them on your every move. Share your progress judiciously and avoid the temptation to over-evangelize to the point of becoming preachy - to succeed people need to find their own motivation for lifestyle changes.

Your Motivation

If asked, most people would like to lead a healthier life and most believe that they should. And when pressed, most agree that health is wealth but yet spend far more time in the pursuit of wealth than health, often to the detriment of the latter.

Motivation intensity, longevity and source will vary vastly from person to person - some will have a health scare that stirs them into action, some will naturally realize it's a good thing, some will have tried before and failed but will try again with the aid of technology. And hopefully some people will read this book and try something with their new-found awareness of what's possible.

I've personally seen people who were largely disinterested in their own well-being find it suddenly and unexpectedly compelling to track their steps when gifted a tracker. Conversely, I have as well seen people who profess to being interested in losing weight but losing interest in the wearable technology when it didn't match their outfit. But this is really an excuse - if you don't like the fashion or aesthetics of a device, but claim to be interested in getting help to achieve your health goals, then try a different form factor. Maybe switch from a visible wrist-based device to an invisible one you clip somewhere out of the way. The technology now comes in so many different guises that only the most obtuse will fail to find one they can tolerate.

How much time and money do you want to invest in well-being? Well it probably depends largely on when you ask the question. Ask a busy person who is generally healthy and they will claim to be too busy to invest time in preventative healthcare. Ask someone who has a health condition or has had a health scare and they will likely be a more attentive audience. If you've grown up exposed to illness, your perspective and value placed on things may be different. I know that the friend of mine with CF who spends the first 90 minutes of every day every morning of her life hooked up to a machine would gladly trade that for the "chore" of spending 15 minutes meditating each day to calm mind and body.

I found it quite insightful to review this survey I received recently from a company that produces a calorie tracking app - clearly they have ideas about what an array of motivations exist and are trying to better understand what motivates their users:

Question - What anticipated reward is most likely to motivate you to improve your health and fitness?
- Feeling generally healthier: physically and mentally
- Living longer or improving (or reducing the impact of) an existing health condition
- Dropping a clothing size
- Getting admiring comments from others
- Romance: pleasing your current partner, getting a new one, or saving a relationship
- Getting positive responses on photos posted on social media
- Performing better in team sports or being able to to do physically-demanding activities
- Performing better at work

Finding Time for Health and Well-Being

Even if you are suitably motivated, equipped with the latest gadgets, have set yourself wellness goals or targets and have even recruited some friends to support your efforts, you may still struggle to achieve your aims. Why? Because undoubtedly, a healthier lifestyle requires time. It's an investment in your future but without a guaranteed payback or visible timeframe, it's not always an easy investment to justify.

In the movie About a Boy, Hugh Grant's character described breaking his life up into segments of time:

> *I find the key is to think of a day as units of time, each unit consisting of no more than thirty minutes. Full hours can be a little bit intimidating and most activities take about half an hour. Taking a bath: one unit, watching countdown: one unit, web-based research: two units, exercising: three units, having my hair carefully disheveled: four units. It's amazing how the day fills up!*

While most of us don't have the luxury of not working that his character had, there is merit in his approach to ensuring we are making use of the time we have and thinking of it as scarce resource with opportunity cost. And realistically don't forget you probably need about one unit a week to manage and monitor everything.

How do you make time? In the spirit of this book, I should advise you that there are plenty of apps about time management that you can consult but it's fundamentally about prioritizing. No matter how busy you are, take a moment to consider how important your health is. By recognizing it's important, you can look at your diary and see 10, 15, 20 minutes a day - everybody has that much time if they really want to. Yes, something else may have to suffer. Yes, it may be hard. Yes, there may be distractions and interruptions which is why it is something that while it's individual, it may be something you need support from others. Could you make half an hour a week in your life if it potentially extended the lifespan or improved the quality of life for you or your loved ones?

One For All The Family

I include loved ones on purpose. While much of the technologies discussed here are for the individual user, many include a family mode - the ability to track vital signs for multiple family members in a single app. Parents who see the benefit of promoting a healthy lifestyle may find technology aids them in communicating this value to the digital natives generation. So if you won't find the time for yourself, would you find it for your childrens' well-being? Changing behavior is difficult and attempts at dramatic changes are more likely to fail if you need to unlearn behaviors and break habits. Many of our good habits are ingrained from childhood and there is a clear opportunity for parents to instill healthy lifestyle habits in children by making monitoring vital signs and well-being a fun family activity.

But just as I describe a scenario of parents using technology to track their kids' well-being and encourage healthy lifestyles, I can easily imagine reverse education where kids show their parents the latest technologies and how to use them - just like the 1980s when kids were the masters showing their parents how VCRs worked.

Time and Time Again

Of all the excuses we dream up to talk ourselves out of healthier living 'lack of time' is at the top of most lists, although the more honest amongst us may just say they'll enjoy life now and worry about it later! But I would propose that finding a few minutes a day to devote to well-being is, indeed, possible. It's a matter of prioritization and habit. It requires discipline, and some days it can be challenging, but the benefits are substantial.

The advent of health and well-being-focused technologies in the last couple of years takes away these lingering excuses around not be able to live a healthier life. Your phone can intelligently and contextually bring to your attention your behaviors/choices and the potential impact on your well-being. The phone and associated accessories are empowering you to take control of your own well-being, on your own terms, in your own home, in your own time. If it's important to you, you will find time. 10 minutes a day on brain relaxation, 10 minutes a day on brain training, 10 minutes a day on recording food or finding healthier options. Build exercise into your day rather than see it as 30 or 90 minutes you have to find.

I'll say it again - putting time aside to look after your health is a big ask. It's a daily imposition of a significant amount of time with what some consider to be no immediate or guaranteed payback. Your view on the relative merits of the time invested probably depends on a few things such as your current health and your close relatives' health. People like instant gratification and quick fixes. Unfortunately, they tend to be very rare and there is very little certainty in life and even less in medicine. That's why I called this book "Your Phone Can Save Your Life" not "Your Phone Will Save Your Life".

Whatever you call it, the ability of technology to remind is vital. You may prefer to call it your "coach" as that sounds more positive than "nag". The variety of options, frequency and media should mean there is a reminder/coach/encouragement level to suit all behavior types. And remember although I'm a big advocate of it as an assistant, the technology we're discussing here is only ever an aid - if you lack commitment, it won't work just because you have an app or an accessory. The Exist Mood Tracking App I mentioned earlier makes a good point as it reminds you to log your day's rating - "technically we don't track your mood, you do!" It does come back to you, not the technology. It's just an aid. Ultimately the technology can only act as a reminder and facilitator.

Patient Engagement/The (Somewhat) Informed Patient

A little learning is a dangerous thing.

- Alexander Pope

Patient engagement is a hot topic in medical circles - Leonard Kish recently called patient engagement "the blockbuster drug" of the century and an increasing amount of engagement, as we have seen, is coming via the once humble mobile phone that is becoming the all-powerful smart hub of our social, entertainment, financial, utilities and now medical information.

The Social Patient

Being unwell was historically a lonely time for people. While the better off were historically cared for at home and only the poor were hospitalized, the standard of care for the less well-off has fallen as specialized care has become more expensive and characterized by hospitals.

We humans are social and curious creatures. For centuries, paternalistic medicine often advocated keeping patients (metaphorically) in the dark - the renowned Hippocrates advised physicians to be economical with the truth to reduce the anxiety of patients. In the 18th century, the physician Thomas Percival wrote that "the life of a sick person can be shortened not only by the acts, but also by the words or manner of a physician."

In the age of information at your fingertips, it may take time for people to adjust to the myriad sources of medical information now available and to discern their quality. But patients can now expect their doctors to be forthcoming with information - the AMA (American Medical Association - not the other use of the acronym, Against Medical Advice!) now recommends: "Withholding medical information from patients without their knowledge or consent is ethically unacceptable." Despite the very personal and individual nature of most illnesses, we are increasingly keen to learn more about our condition(s), and about how others have coped with similar complaints in the hopes of learning from them. A generation of people used to being able to look up anything on the Internet is consumerizing medicine as well as medicalizing consumerism.

The first generation of medicine on the internet was the rather hit-and-miss experience of looking up symptoms on the internet. As one of the most common uses of the Internet, it's no surprise that many companies have stepped in to bring more order to symptom searches - now you have dedicated curated health information surfacing when you search Google for health terms as well as respected sites like WebMD (which sees 12.5m visitors per month) and dedicated communities for pretty much every imaginable ailment.

Some of the most interesting apps in this area are built around these web sites to offer support, information or tracking of symptoms.

- Patients Like Me claims over 350,000 members tracking over 2,500 conditions. The site enables people to create a free profile with the aim of sharing experiences of illnesses, with the additional desire of supporting research. Their corporate goals "envision a future where every patient benefits from the collective experience of all, and where the risk and reward of each possible choice is transparent and known." The site has recently signed a deal with the FDA to determine how patient-reported data can give new insights into drug safety - more on that later. PLM users can record symptoms, quality of life, lab results, treatments and hospitalizations as well as discussing their experiences in forums with similar users or choose to share their data with researchers. The app allows you to update your current mood or symptoms and see timeline updates from users you've chosen to follow.

- Flaredown is a service designed to assist sufferers of Chronic conditions to document and better understand their conditions over time. Daily, you log your condition level, each symptom level as well as what medication you took along with a note on any activities you undertook. Progressively, this provides a graphical view that can help you understand changes over time, as well as identify factors that exacerbate or ameliorate your condition(s).

- Founded by the former Chief Health Strategist at Google, smartpatients.com is a start-up online community aimed at motivated patients, who want to understand more about their condition, share their experiences and search for clinical trials that may be relevant to them. The site is free to patients and caregivers, and makes its money by selling anonymized information to the pharmaceutical and research industries.

- Iodine is a medications-centered site containing pharmacists explanations of medications combined with patient reviews and ratings. Site members are encouraged to learn about drugs, their benefits and side effects, as well as offering side by side comparisons of alternatives. Users rate medicines on a three-point scale - was it worth it, did it work and was it a hassle. For people doing a lot of research on their condition on the web, it offers a handy add on (a "Chrome extension") for your web browser that automatically highlights medical terms on other web sites and provides pop-up information from Iodine in the context of the page you're looking at.

Reviewing the Medical Profession

One of the most common types of sites on the internet is review sites (Yelp, Trip Advisor, etc.) so it was probably inevitable that rate my doctor type sites and mobile apps would emerge such as healthgrades.com. While obviously it is important to have faith in your medical professional, and doctors should be encouraged to treat their patients with respect, it is important to note that there are significant challenges unique to this sector in terms of ratings as patients may not be in a position to accurately assess their doctor's expertise objectively. Patients who do not agree with a perfectly valid medical opinion may give a low rating, or people who were denied access to a medicine they desired may vent their frustration on these sites.

While there are now many resources such as those discussed above available for people to better understand and even manage chronic illnesses, let's return to the focus of this book which is more on prevention.

Improving Research?

Even though the primary purpose of technology-enabled patient communities is the exchange of information among sufferers, it will be interesting to see what impact the rise of patient sites and mobile data recording has on the previously closed world of pharmaceutical research. Patient communities may be able to influence trial design, highlight previously relevant findings that the trial owners may not be aware of and to direct studies more towards what matters to patients, as this is surprisingly regularly quite far down the priority for a trial.

It may also help to influence an end to the practice of drugs trials that compare new drugs to a placebo rather than the current best available treatments - a practice that benefits drug companies more than patients. Any improvement in the efficacy and efficiency of trials may help better direct the spending of industry funding for the widest possible benefit.

It seems likely that major patient communities facilitated by technology will provide a better means to engage patients in testing and capture of on-going feedback on drug efficacy. There have been efforts before such as the 2008 EU and the 2009 NHS initiatives to involve the public more through the web sites Patientpartner-europe.eu and invo.org.uk but the announcement that the FDA is partnering with Patients Like Me brings a scale to these efforts that is very promising. The PatientsLikeMe and FDA research collaboration will seek to determine how patient-reported data can give new insights into drug safety and give a more complete picture about a drug's safety by changing post-launch surveillance for drugs. This will augment the clinical trials data which may only include the experience of several hundred or at most several thousand patients thus making it possible to uncover patient impacts that aren't evident in trials.

While on the one hand it is enticing to think of improvements in research by increased patient involvement and greater transparency; on the other hand, patient power, individual desperation and a media hunger for unlikely dramatic breakthroughs must be managed to ensure that rigorous trial procedures are not abandoned to the detriment of evidence-based medicine. Pharmaceutical company involvement, either explicit or unstated, with patient groups may lead to extensive "pester power" for unproven and expensive drugs to shortcut the lengthy route to market before efficacy and safety are convincingly established. Direct to consumer drug advertising that is normal in the US, but banned in other countries, might subtly enter into European culture through social media and other non-traditional channels, marking a surreptitious shift in medical communications and industry balance of power.

Facilitating Trials

Trials are essential to progress but are expensive, time consuming and difficult to setup. Apple's ResearchKit is an open source software framework that makes it easier for researchers and developers to create apps for medical studies - the company hopes to make it simpler for universities and research hospitals to find participants for medical trials and studies by making it far easier to conduct medical trials, which are a key basis of evidence-based medicine. By providing much of the "plumbing" required to build apps for research projects, Apple may be enabling researchers to focus on solving problems rather than grappling with the logistics of finding and collecting data.

"Numbers are everything. The more people who contribute their data, the bigger the numbers, the truer the representation of a population, and the more powerful the results. A research platform that allows large amounts of data to be collected and shared — that can only be a positive thing for medical research." Dr. Eduardo Sanchez, American Heart Association

Summoning Help

Another innovative use of mobile technology to help save other people's lives is the GoodSAM app. We've all seen the dramatic movie scenes with "Is there a Doctor on the plane?" announcements but in everyday life when people experience medical crises, as they wait for an ambulance, there may be a trained first responder nearby who is available to help but unaware of the problem.

People interested in availing of the GoodSAM service simply download the Alerter app and in the event of an emergency, use the app to call the emergency services. At the same time, the app will search for GoodSAM Responders - those with medical training who are willing to give potentially life-saving interventions before the arrival of emergency services using a crowd-sourced database of public defibrillators (machines which use an electric charge to restart a heart in the event of a cardiac arrest). Keep in mind that even with the best response times of an ambulance, it's critical for survival to receive cardiopulmonary resuscitation (CPR - chest compressions and rescue breaths) and defibrillation in the first three to four minutes after an event. If an defibrillator is used within two minutes, there is an 80% chance that the victim will survive.

This app raises many questions about indemnity/liability and risk but some jurisdictions already have good samaritan legislation that is probably relevant. GoodSAM require volunteers to upload evidence of their qualifications and provide a code of conduct intended to avert potential legal issues. But just like the disruptive technologies in other industries that have challenged legislative frameworks (Uber, AirBnB), apps like GoodSam will push legislators into uncharted territory.

Your Directives?

I've written a lot in this book about mobile technology's role in saving, extending or improving life but there is an inevitable conclusion for us all. We don't know when or how it will happen, of course, but there may be medical decisions to be made at this difficult time. End-of-life care preference is an understandably sensitive subject. It is not a topic that a lot of people are comfortable talking about but tends to rise to the top of the agenda as people age or are diagnosed with life threatening conditions. However, for people caught in emergency or trauma situations, there can be uncertainty about their wishes for such eventualities if for example they are suddenly left too injured or ill to communicate preferences about treatment.

With Apple Health in iOS 8, Apple introduced a feature where you can choose to make your blood group, medical conditions, allergies and medications available even when your phone screen is locked. It can also show your organ donation preferences, negating the need to procure a separate organ donor card as a barrier to recording your desires, should the need to know your intentions arise. Apple have been unusually candid that they have big plans for the health arena so I'm sure we'll see many more health features in future iPhones, Apple Watch and Apps.

Going further than Apple Health's emergency information display, an app called MyDirectives enables people to record their own emergency medical care plan which can be accessed by family and doctors in a time of need. Physicians may decide unwittingly to act against your wishes if they do not know them. I appreciate that many people struggle to put their ICE (In Case of Emergency) contact in their phones, and few have thoughts of Do Not Resuscitate (DNR) orders or Physician Orders for Life-Sustaining Treatment (POLST) but that's what MyDirectives is designed for. It includes sections for your priorities, treatment decisions as well as your designated agents and relatives.

Saving Others

So far I've talked primarily about how mobile technology might help to improve or extend your own well-being. This may place me (or you if you adopt any of my recommendations) at risk of accusations of selfishness for an over-obsessive or self-indulgent focus. So I want to briefly outline how the technology now packed into your phone might also help other people. Aside of course from the enormous societal benefits of your improved health reducing the burden on the health service and perhaps resulting in quicker access for others to specialists, there are other ways that your pocket computing power can assist the wider good if appropriately channeled. So whether this book has helped you to decide to do something about your own well-being or not, maybe consider if you want to contribute to that of others or to the greater good.

Your Phone can Save other People's Lives in at least two different ways - donating your computing power to researchers, and/or contributing information anonymously.

Distributed Computing

As we've noted several times, the processing power of smartphones is increasing at a dramatic pace - outstripping the famous Moore's Law that predicts the doubling of computing power every 18 months. The iPhone 4 more processing power than a decade old supercomputer and the iPhone 6 has many times more power again. With Google activating over 100,000 Android devices per hour and Apple selling 34,000 iPhones per hour, there are now more far more mobile computing devices in the world than people. However, typically these powerful processing units lie nearly dormant for approximately 8 hours a day as we sleep, creating a combined untapped wealth of computing power.

Several apps now exist that break up some of the world's largest outstanding computational challenges into small pieces which are sent to individual phones which work on the problem overnight and then send the completed data back to the project to be combined into the overall analysis. Both Sony (Folding@Home) which powers research projects in collaboration with Stanford and HTC (Power to Give) allow you to select what projects you support and only operate when your phone is plugged in and operating via WiFi. By harnessing the combined distributed computing power of the world's smartphones, perhaps some project which does not get time allocations on university supercomputers will help scientists make progress.

Chapter 10:
Future Doctors & Future Patients

No industry is immune and no occupation is safe. All of us need
to begin to think in terms of our own inner strengths, our
resilience and resourcefulness, our capacity to adapt.
- Stephen Pressfield

Recent years have seen Industries that previously seemed
unchangeable being rapidly up-ended as web and mobile
technologies mature and move in with new forms of disruption -
accommodation, taxi services and television to name but a few
(via Airbnb, Uber and Netflix respectively) have seen decades old
business models challenged, with deeply entrenched incumbents
scrambling to react to an exodus of customers to the upstart
organizations that didn't exist just a couple of years ago. The
generation who have grown up with on-demand everything will
not accept waiting for doctor's appointments and will fully expect
reviews of healthcare to play a part in maintaining quality and
making it transparent.

Healthcare is an industry unlike any other, but its sensitive
position and the need for great care in introducing change
doesn't mean we should miss opportunities for genuine
improvement. Silicon Valley often gets criticized for backing too
many photo-sharing apps and solving too many first-world
problems, like having underwear delivered to your doorstep in an
hour. Digital Health is anything but this kind of sector and the
first half of 2015 saw over $1bn invested in health-related
startups, which shows that investors believe healthcare is now at
a tipping point with the gates opening to outsiders for the first
time.

It's going to be a dramatic shift for the medical industry, but as I've mentioned, virtually every industry faces seismic shifts and by my reckoning, healthcare is overdue. While they are happening, these changes can be painful for those involved in adjusting to upheaval and alterations in expectations and responsibilities. But despite some missteps along the way, the period of change should result in the emergence of a stronger, leaner industry/sector. With one as crucial as health, we need to get this right, both in human and in financial terms. Let's be clear though, it's not just about changing medical professionals - the new order of healthcare places an unprecedented degree of capability, and therefore responsibility, firmly on patients.

Wide-Ranging Impacts

Industries that fail to adapt and adopt new technologies will come under huge pressures in the coming years and the once seemingly impregnable world of healthcare will not survive untouched in its current form. Newly informed patients will be empowered and digital natives will instinctively turn to their phones in times of trouble. The General Practitioner in future years may see her surgery waiting room empty as patients seek advice from online doctors for many of the most common ailments. Yet we don't want to risk the intrinsically human art of medicine by not recognizing the value, both social and medical, of face to face consultations.

The impact of technology is already being felt in the wellness sector - industry stalwart Weight Watchers blamed a significant portion of its 78% share drop in 3 years on customers moving to apps instead of paying to attend WW sessions, as noted by Weight Watchers Chief Financial Officer Nicholas Hotchkin who said at an investor conference "We were particularly susceptible to the proliferation of free apps and activity monitors."

There will be winners and losers along the way in this revolution. Ultimately, we should all win, but at times it may seem like we're going backwards as different stakeholders move at varying paces and entrenched interests seek to protect privileged or traditional positions. Ownership of the future of healthcare falls between many vested interests. Technologists who don't appreciate the practice of medicine, patients who are short-termist, prone to over-react and misinterpret information, doctors who aren't able to keep pace with developments or be open to change, pharmaceutical giants, insurance companies and private hospitals acting in the best interests of their bottom line where patients are more important to them than people. And, of course, Governments disinterested in any program that doesn't guarantee improvements in a timeframe shorter than the next election. This complex web of stakeholders will take time to readjust to new realities.

The majority of practicing doctors today left medical school at a time when smartphones didn't exist and were not trained to expect empowered patients who could monitor their own vital signs.

If you don't yet see the impact of new technologies on the frontlines of healthcare, before you blame intransigent doctors, consider that the App Store has only really been with us for just 7 years and the iPad only 5.

Looking 5 or 10 years ahead, the questions we see now will have long been answered. As with the advent of any momentous change, there are still many unknowns to consider as we decide if and how we want to assimilate these technologies into our lives:

- Will it create a generation of hypochondriacs or more appropriately termed cyberchondriacs?
- What about the impact on the current generation of doctors?
- Are people least likely to benefit the most likely to use technology?
- Will we lose the human touch from healthcare

The gold-rush to a newly democratized healthcare sector will see new entrants in the market, and some existing players fall by the wayside. Asked to name the leading health companies in the world, most people would probably mention the likes of GlaxoSmithKline or Pfizer. These pharmaceutical giants have undoubtedly saved the lives of countless people, as well as improved the lives of millions more by giving them relief from physical or psychological symptoms. Yet in years to come, anybody asked to name the leading health companies in the world may well say "Google" or "Apple". Strange as it may sound now, these Internet and Mobile giants are emerging as key players in forming and facilitating the future of healthcare. If the 1900s saw the emergence of medicines coming to the forefront, the 2000s maybe remembered first for the rise to prominence of technology-enhanced monitoring and care, ahead of the expected dividend of research into genetics (our DNA) and microbiomics (the trillion or so bacteria that live in and on you in a complex symbiotic relationship we don't yet fully understand).

Great Technology is Invisible

Only very few people will be interested in actively managing their well-being via multiple apps and sensors. And that's the way it should be. The technology exists to monitor us without requiring frequent input and while it currently requires considerable user attention to monitor your health, the effort required will rapidly diminish as the technology improves and fades into the background.

While journalists writing about the emergence of more personal and portable technologies that underpin the changing landscape of healthcare today love to label it as "wearable" technology, that is, in fact, a bit of a misnomer. The focus should not be on the technology - it's not about the devices and whether they are attached to us or simply about information conveyed to our smartphone - it's about the life-improving actions these technologies can enable or encourage. And it's about the human interactions and behaviors that these technologies will revolutionize - changing how we consume medical care and making sure medical care doesn't consume us.

Future Doctors

"We look for medicine to be an orderly field of knowledge and procedure. But it is not. It is an imperfect science, an enterprise of constantly changing knowledge, uncertain information, fallible individuals, and at the same time lives on the line. There is science in what we do, yes, but also habit, intuition, and sometimes plain old guessing. The gap between what we know and what we aim for persists. And this gap complicates everything we do."

— Atul Gawande, Complications: A Surgeon's Notes on an Imperfect Science

Going to a doctor's surgery when you're ill is not always easy. It may be the time you least feel like going out, it may require waiting for an appointment and more often than not results only in a routine prescription. While having a professional check you over and give you the all clear that it's nothing more serious than a sore throat that will be gone by the weekend is reassuring, it is also highly inefficient. But we must remember that doctors develop a unique ability to diagnose. And it's not just about the hard data. It involves body language, subtle observation and even intuition. The technology is not yet anywhere near advanced enough to start replacing those skills. Where self-monitoring technology can help most is in supporting awareness. And highlighting areas for professional or clinical investigation before they would otherwise become apparent.

Consider a future scenario: Before you even notice you're not feeling 100%, your phone tells you it has detected a slight elevation in your heart rate and your temperature, as well as your breathing rate. It asks you if you're feeling ok and suggests you consult your online nurse service by video call. You agree and within moments, you're sitting looking at a nurse on the screen, who has access to your health data. You confirm you're feeling like you're maybe coming down with a cold and slight sore throat. The nurse suggests a mild antibiotic given your history of sore throats, and recommends you take things easy for a few days and she'll be in touch if you don't improve. She notes that your blood pressure and weight are stable and congratulates you for keeping active in recent months. A final reminder that you should get in touch if you don't feel better within 48 hours or develop any other symptoms. Two more button presses and the next two things on your list are done - your boss just got an email confirming your absence for the next two days, and your pharmacy got an order to deliver the prescription to you in the next two hours. And all the costs of this was covered by your annual medical subscription and the details are recorded in your online medical record, which is available to your physician who is alerted that you had a consult.

In another scenario, you might notice a tightness in your chest, and consult a physician via an app. It's the weekend so your normal doctor isn't available but you're slightly worried. The video doctor asks you to place the Bluetooth stethoscope your insurer provided on your chest and she listens remotely. Not happy with the result, she suggests you should come in to the clinic, and offers to send an Uber car to get you. You say you'll make your own way and the directions to the nearest suitable clinic pop up on your phone, along with a confirmed appointment for the next morning.

For anyone worried that the scenarios above are impersonal, consider that the emphasis on a personal relationship with a doctor is not always the case - you don't plan when you're going to be sick and if your doctor isn't available, you will gladly take an appointment with a locum doctor. Let's be clear that I am in no way advocating a wholesale removal of human interaction from medical practice. If you've seen the movie Up in the Air, you'll recall George Clooney's reaction to being replaced by a video call. But if routine matters can be handled more efficiently by these kinds of remote services, then my belief is that doctors can devote more personal time to the people who need it most.

When you do still visit a doctor's clinic, the data you've collected via your mobile will be available to your physician if you've chosen to share it with them. The data-driven nature of consultations may result in a change of layout in clinical rooms as discussion of the data, trends and insights become central as a replacement for the rather vague "history" based on memory and approximations. But patients do not want doctors looking at the screen instead of them - I foresee a change in the layout of doctor surgeries where larger screens enable joint review of data and images. Just like Catholic priests turned to face the congregation for mass in 1964, doctors must remove barriers from their patient interactions. And doctors will rightly have little respect for patients trying to look up PLM or Iodine every time a doctor mentions a possible drug.

It is important to consider how the role of doctor will evolve in this new healthcare landscape. They will likely spend a larger proportion of time spent as a consultant not a physician and as a data analyst not just a test-requester. They must not become monitors who merely react to alarms from systems warning about a change in patient data nor merely an overseer of patient compliance.

Our current interactions with the health system in the coming years will seem as bizarre as explaining to today's online generation that pictures were once taken on chemical film that had to be sent away before you could see the photos, TV shows could only be watched when they were scheduled and movies were on "tapes" you had to rewind before bringing them back to video stores to avoid fines. Just as we now regard historical medical practices as barbaric and ignorant, not long from now, some of our current norms will be seen just as similarly archaic and arcane.

The American Medical Association (AMA) estimates that 70% of doctor office visits *could* have been provided as effectively remotely - from a medical standpoint, if not a social one. But as remote visits become the norm, this will doubtless impact the availability and economics of surgeries. And where will the social element come from - will it be from Online support groups such as PatientsLikeMe?

Apps for Doctors

Continuing Professional Development (CPD) is a vital part of many high skill sectors, perhaps none more so than the medical profession. The pace of change, progress due to new trials, research or technology and the evolution of our understanding of a range of illnesses mean that the state of medicine during a doctor's 40 year career may be vastly different from that at the start of medical school. And I for one am keen that my caregivers are always as up to date as they can be. The statistic from the US Department of Labor that 65% of school-goers today will be in careers that don't exist yet only serves to illustrate the pace of change that we now face.

It is inevitable that much of the CPD for doctors will move online and onto mobile, just as with other disciplines. All of what we've talked about so far has been patient-centric. And that's the intended focus of the book. But it's worth noting the growing number of apps being created to help doctors - apps created for doctors, and in many cases, by doctors. So the next time you visit your doctor and she's looking intently at her phone, she may be looking at an app that helps find a solution for you - so don't get offended too quickly! For the curious, some of the most popular apps that doctors have access to are outlined here. While most users are used to free apps, and maybe the occasional in app purchase, apps aimed at doctors frequently follow a different business model - They are often subscription-based with annual subscriptions that combined would total over $760 for the most popular apps. This does however give a degree of comfort about the quality of the material they include. Some do have an amount of free content or offer patient versions, but be warned that most of the information in these apps is far beyond the comprehension of most non-professional users and may simply end up confusing any lay person trying to use them.

- Medscape from WebMD has a million registered users and is aimed at physicians, medical students, nurses and other healthcare professionals The app is available for free and is open to consumers. It offers comprehensives Medical News, Drug Information, coverage of 4,400+ diseases and conditions as well as over 100 medical calculators covering formulas, scales, and classifications along with drug dosing calculators. Offline access within the app means you don't have to be online to use it, which is useful as some hospitals and clinics lack WiFi.

- Another of the best known general physician reference apps, Epocrates claim that 50% of US doctors use their app, with over 1 million healthcare professionals signed up worldwide. A free version includes a large amounts of health information, with a paid upgrade for professionals offering additional features and information. Its reference materials include drug interactions, pill identification, research updates, treatments for infectious diseases, and a Directory for referrals. It also includes over 40 calculation tools from things as common as BMI, to highly specialized formulae, such as the Parkland formula that is used when treating burns patients.

- Well-established as an online resource, UpToDate is positioned as a clinical decision support resource with evidence-based information – including drug topics and treatment recommendations. Conducting research with UpToDate is recognized as Continuing Medical Education for doctors in several countries. Available by subscription for doctors, consumers or patients can also choose to subscribe for as little as a week if they want access to the same information resources as doctors. In addition, it provides over 1,500 articles that clinicians can review with patients in the exam room, print out as handouts, or send via email.

- Isabel is a diagnosis app to help clinicians broaden their differential diagnosis and assist in cases where clinicians that may have diagnostic doubt or want reassurance on a particular diagnostic conclusion. It was founded by a family whose daughter was misdiagnosed, and prompts doctors to think of possible alternative causes based on the presenting symptoms. It has the ability to handle natural language / free text and is intended to act as a reminder to the physician - decision making is still left to the physician. A patient-friendly version called Isabel Symptom Checker is available intended for patients to help better inform them when talking to their doctor.

- Sometimes referred to as LinkedIn for doctors, Doximity is the largest medical professional network in the US, with over 50% of physicians as members. As well as personal profile listings, it offers physicians tools for HIPAA[2]-secure communication and Continuing Medical Education credits for reading news articles as well as the all-important job seeking facilities.

---

[2] HIPAA is the US Federal Health Insurance Portability and Accountability Act of 1996. The primary goal of the law is to make it easier for people to keep health insurance, protect the confidentiality and security of healthcare information and help the healthcare industry control administrative costs.

- Figure 1 is an app that aims to create a knowledge sharing community for doctors, nurses, medical students, and other healthcare professionals to discuss and share real-world medical cases. Featuring anonymized patient cases (via both automatic face blocking and a manual blocking tool), it allows members to view thousands of clinical cases organized by anatomy area and specialty including photos, X-Rays, MRIs, CAT scans and ECGs. Boasting over 500,000 downloads from more than 100 countries worldwide and, as of September 2015, over 1 billion views of cases, it includes a paging feature, where healthcare professionals can virtually "page" a network of specialists for fast feedback on clinical cases that they upload, opening the opportunity to explore medical cases previously unique to certain parts of the globe. I've seen Figure 1 described as "Instagram for Doctors" - but having had a look, I can warn you that the images are not the type usually shared on Instagram!

- Appscript is a platform that helps doctors select appropriate consumer mobile apps and accessories to recommend to patients. It has curated and categorized thousands of mobile healthcare apps as well as hundreds of connected devices. Doctors can use it to send recommendations directly to their patients' phones. It really does enable doctors to prescribe apps alongside or instead of medicine.

How to Keep Up

Medicine is already an information intensive industry and its dependence on data and analysis may accelerate faster than any other sector in the coming years. As the mysteries of the 21,000 or so human genes are decoded, we are generating massive amounts of data - a single human genome is about 100 gigabytes in its raw data format. Specialist services to store this data is now available from both Google or Amazon's cloud storage services for less than $5 per month. Scientists conducting studies comparing genetic data across large groups are now facing quantities of data that run to petabytes (a petabyte is 1 million gigabytes) and just as Wall Street competed with Silicon Valley in the 1990s for mathematical talent, Medicine will require ever more experts in data analysis and algorithms in the coming years to help doctors extract relevant information from the mind-boggling amount of data being created and uncovered.

And in case you thought that the decoding of the human genome was the end of the avalanche of data, beyond our genetic data, much research attention is now shifting to understanding our microbiome - looking at the DNA of the 100 trillion microscopic organisms we share our bodies with but know very little about. Keeping up with the developments and information that will flow from analyzing, cross referencing and understanding this data will challenge future doctors' capabilities to keep abreast of current best practice more than ever before.

Thankfully Doctors will have some of the world's most powerful technology to assist them wade through all of this data - IBM has set about enhancing its super-computer "Watson" with medical diagnostic features, based on assimilating and analyzing vast quantities of medical knowledge. But the aim is not to replace doctors: Rob Merkel, who leads IBM Watson's health group, said "We're not advocating that Watson replace physicians. We are advocating that Watson does a lot of reading on behalf of physicians and provides them with timely insights."

Between the data now stored on my phone and in the cloud storage that my phone has instant access to, I have captured vast quantities of data about my body and its history. Some of what I and my phone knows a doctor could know and fill in many of the gaps by checking my record. But the DNA-level knowledge I can access via my phone since I had my genes decoded is information they can't know or infer from their experience. And they may not even be equipped to interpret it - there may not have been any humans in the world with their DNA decoded when they were in medical school. Yet my DNA report contains pharmacogenomic (genetic sensitivity to drugs) information that is potentially vital to my well-being. I have a genetic disposition to a stronger than normal reaction to blood thinners for example. In years gone by, it was unthinkable that I could know such a fact before my doctor - now I am simply keen that any medical professional treating me has access to this information to assist in their decision making. But what does this shift in information access mean for the doctor-patient relationship?

In his book "Automate This: How Algorithms Came to Rule Our World", Christopher Steiner describes how he sees algorithms benefiting medicine: *"imagine a doctor who will always be convenient and available, know all of your strengths and weaknesses, know every single risk factor your past conditions might signal, know your complete medical history, know the medical history of the last three generations of your family, never make a careless mistake or write an incorrect prescription, always be up to date on every new treatment and medical discovery, never fall into bad habits, know by heart each one of your baselines measurements: pulse, cholesterol, weight, blood pressure, lung capacity, bone density and past injuries, monitor you at all times, always be searching for the hint of a problem, be it at heart tick, or creeping blood pressure increase, a cholesterol surge or even trace changes in the air you expel which could indicate early stage cancer. There exists no human doctor who can do these things - an algorithm can and will do all of them. The evidence in favour of algorithms at the bedside is piling up. The hospitals that use algorithms in their standard processes, have fewer complications, more correct initial diagnoses, lower fatality rates and yes, lower costs."*

The Doctor-Patient Relationship

"Declare the past, diagnose the present, foretell the future."

— Hippocrates

The good physician treats the disease; the great physician treats the patient who has the disease.

- William Osler

Many medical professionals fear that this revolution will trivialize medicine but, in my view, nothing could be further from the truth. These developments open the potential for medical professionals to channel their talents into higher level contributions and have more informed conversations with their patients. I for one would be heartened to think that my GP can augment his knowledge and experience with access to a super-computer that can assess my case against all accumulated medical knowledge in the world. Bear in mind that if a doctor were to read for 30 hours a day, every day, they could not keep up with all published medical research.

The ancient Greek physician Hippocrates, who has had a lasting impact on medical thinking, believed in concealing the patient's condition from them. This deep seated paternalism is well documented by authors such as Topol and Katz and has been defended until recently by the medical bodies such as the AMA. Patients generally do and should trust those people trained to look after them. But they should also question them, and as is often the case, look for a second opinion. It would be naive to think that a Google search can replace a minimum of 8 years of medical school tuition, but it's equally naive to think that a single doctor cannot benefit from accessing a database of combined medical knowledge as well as up to date information - much will have changed since the doctor left school. And while day to day experience may be a great teacher, it cannot account for the breadth of knowledge accumulated on a daily basis worldwide.

Pocket Triage

Some services, interactions and relationships are harder to move online than others. But there are probably very few things that won't move at least somewhat online in the future. As communication, entertainment, shopping and banking have succumbed progressively to the march of internet and smartphone convenience, online medical care is now too becoming a viable option in a widening number of circumstances. Whether it's more efficient access to information, appointments or virtual consultations, there is now a mobile option to deliver convenience for the on-demand generation.

People have increasingly relied on web searches in recent years for medical information, to the point where most surveys show that about 70% of people have at some point turned to Google for clues about their symptoms. But in most cases, whatever information they gained has led to a conventional doctor or clinic visit, supplemented with questions to their physician based on their newly gleaned web results.

Finding a doctor and making an appointment to see them was previously likely to be a lengthy exercise. Now with services such as Zocdoc, you can search for a doctor in your locality that specializes in your required medical condition, see their appointment availability for the next three days and click to make an appointment - it is as easy booking a doctor's appointment as popular app OpenTable makes finding a restaurant. And if you want to shop around for treatment costs before you want speak to a doctor, take guroo.com as an example This lets you enter your condition and see what the pricing for a procedure or treatment bundle is in your area, as well as a comparison to national averages.

An App a Day Keeps the Doctor Away

House calls, which accounted for 40% of all doctor visits in 1930, represented less than 1% by 1980 as physicians found it far more efficient to have people come to them in their clinics. Yet a majority of visits to doctors' surgeries are objectively unnecessary. Most people know what is wrong with them in advance of the "diagnosis" and have a clear preconception of what they want as a result of the visit, often right down to the specific pill they want to see prescribed.

There is an ever growing number of virtual doctor services vying for space on your phone, but here's a summary of some of the leading ones and the features now within the grasp of your smartphone. They range from symptom checkers to help you decide if you need to see a doctor right up to full video consultations with doctors. Note that due to varying regulations, all of the apps listed here may not be available in all jurisdictions and some other services such as Heal, Pager and True North currently operate only in very limited catchment areas. Even if that's the case, watch out for similar functionality coming soon and keep in mind that in the very near future the notion of States banning video consultations with doctors will seem as old fashioned as someone insisting you rent a DVD instead of watching Netflix.

- A subscription service (currently £4.99 per month in the UK or €7.99 in Ireland) Babylon offers on-demand video call consultations with certified doctors. The subscription model offers unlimited consultations or you can choose a Pay As You Go model for £29 per session after a free trial. Patients can submit text questions to the service, or upload images for a professional opinion. Babylon also integrates and monitors data from other services or accessories so you have a one-stop-shop for your well-being and the doctor providing your consultation can see your latest steps, weight, sleep, blood pressure, heart rate and other metrics. A mail-in service is also available within the app for you to order home lab test kits. You can purchase tests for cholesterol, kidney function, liver function and blood tests that are delivered to your home. You take the test as instructed and post it back. You receive your results by email and in the app, and Babylon will advise you if any of the results require further investigation.

- Your.MD Symptom Checker offers personal health information on illnesses with content provided by the NHS. Accepting simple voice descriptions of what's troubling you, the symptom checker tries to figure out what might be wrong with you with follow-on questions and then displays information on up to five potential conditions or illnesses, along with how to avoid, manage or treat them. It will advise on whether you should go see a doctor or call an ambulance.

- Dr on Demand (not surprisingly based on the name) offers video sessions with qualified board-certified physicians and psychologists! Charged on a per visit or session basis (currently starting at $40 for physicians, $50 for psychologists) the aim of this app is to diagnose and treat most common medical conditions. As a differentiator, it has also started to offer specialist lactation consultations and basic mental health care - including consultations to address issues such as stress, anxiety, relationship issues and depression.

- GrandRounds is a service that enables you to seek a physician appointment or a second opinion via an app. Designed to connect patients with world-leading specialists in their particular condition, GrandRounds promises to make access to specialized care easier to find.

- iTriage allows you to search health-related symptoms while offline, review potential causes and then find the most appropriate treatment, health facility or doctor. It was created by two ER doctors and draws on medical content reviewed by Harvard Medical School. With over 12 million downloads, it is among the most popular Health Apps. Starting with a visually driven symptom checker, it also features directories of Doctor and Health Facilities such as nearest hospital/emergency department, clinics, pharmacy, doctor, imaging center, mental health clinic, substance abuse clinic, and community health centres complete with average wait times and direct online appointment setting with some facilities.

- Walgreens has partnered with another online provider MD Live to add smartphone-based consultations to its app. This provides an interesting combination of a big consumer brand with massive reach and a new approach to medical care delivery with online consultations. With up to 35 million Walgreens app users, it may point towards a future when telemedicine become your primary first go-to doctor? At $49 per "visit", the cost is comparable to co-pay levels many insurance companies already impose. And the MDLive App has even added a photo of a virtual waiting room in case you're nostalgic while waiting to be connected to your virtual doctor.

- In some states in the US, a service called Cellscope is available for people concerned about ear infections. People can order a small attachment for their phone that turns it into a functioning Otoscope, the device doctor's use to look into your ear. The output of the scope is relayed to a doctor who views the video online and lets the patient know if it's anything to be worried about.

- ZipDrug is a dedicated prescription medicine delivery service that enables you have electronically issued prescriptions delivered to you. Simply place your order via the app and a messenger will deliver your prescription to you. Currently only available in Manhattan, the couriers are trained in HIPAA and special handling and the app provides notifications when refills are due.

Virtual Visits in Context

When considering the attractiveness of online doctor services, it is important to consider the alternatives and the context. I would say that if a video call is not as good as a face to face visit, it is still better than an unmediated review of questionable data sources a patient may find on the Internet and the resulting misguided self-diagnosis that doctors may face if they don't embrace virtual visits.

In the words of well-known commentator health technologies Dr. Joseph Kvedar of Partners HealthCare "We have found, over and over again, that with a healthy, pre-existing doctor/patient relationship, virtual care is a boon and actually strengthens that rapport, because the convenience of virtual care is seen as an extension of the relationship. For example, patients can perceive it as a bonus or advantage.

In his book "The Patient Will See You Know", renowned medical technology expert Dr Eric Topol pointed out that the "smartphone is just a pipe, a conduit of flowing data. On either end of it are intelligent human beings who are ready to assume quite different roles from what the history of medicine has established. He emphasizes the differentiating capabilities of doctors - having an exceptional base of knowledge and judgment to contextualize the patients information while at the same time providing empathy, inspiration and support for the individual to stay health or get healthy.

With average wait time to see a physician of 2½ weeks in the US (according to CNN in August 2014), all of these apps have in common a shift towards on-demand consultations, available 24-7 to patients regardless of their location. People will most likely turn to these services in urgent or out of hours or follow-up scenarios where visiting a doctor is not convenient and the patient may not perceive the need for repeat visit. And if they are happy with the service in these circumstances, they may continue to use it in future. It's also worth noting that many developed nations are facing current or imminent shortages of doctors and nurses. Switzerland could see 75% of their general practitioners retire by 2025 while Germany may have to replace more than 50,000 doctors, including around 23,000 GPs, by only 2020. This lack of resources creates a risk of reduction in access to primary care and an inefficient utilization of limited healthcare budgets. This will prompt debate about the roles and responsibilities of individuals, employers and ultimately the state in population health but may provide a pull factor to the push factor of a tech-savvy generation of health users. Similarly, the WHO states there is a worldwide shortage of doctors. So, even if people are somewhat hesitant about virtual or remote consultations, it is highly likely that mobile access will be the first point of triage for many people in the years to come.

For doctors and practices seeking to embrace technology and cater to patients seeking the convenience of remote consultations, several off-the-shelf solutions are now available. Start-ups such as Fruitstreet.com give Doctors a turnkey set of software components, including a mobile app to offer their patients tele-visits, monitor their vitals and collect payments. This means that non-technically savvy and even small practices can benefit from HIPAA compliant technologies.

Bring your Own D...

There's been a trend in the corporate world called BYOD - Bring Your Own Device. This refers to the increase in people choosing their own smartphone or tablet device for work purposes rather than being supplied with a device, as was the way. This has presented challenges to IT departments in terms of device management, systems compatibility and of course security. Just as the BYOD phenomenon has turned corporate policies on their head in a few short years, so too will hospitals and health services have to look at the implications for their policies, procedures and processes.

In the coming years in the medical space, BYOD will become Bring Your Own Data. For years, it was standard practice if visiting a doctor to bring a small urine sample in a plastic bottle. Now you can conduct the test yourself at home and send them the result. In the case of a definitive Urinary Tract Infection (UTI) result for example, why visit a doctor if there are no other issues or symptoms? Send them the sample result, have a short video conference, then have the doctor electronically prescribe the medicine.

Already my father brings a weekly record of his blood pressure on his bi-annual visit to his cardiologist. This gives such a better picture of on-going well-being than just having the pressure checked twice a year by the doctor during the visit. As norms change in the next few years, I can imagine the look of horror on a doctor's face in years to come if a patient were to show up without detailed data on their vital signs.

For a doctor conducting a video call, they can use both their judgement but also have the camera pointed at the patient send them breathing and heart rate data. If they are worried about something, then of course they should summon the patient for a face to face visit. As an additional benefit of the technology in certain cases, perhaps the ease of access and the distance created by mobile consultations can help overcome patients' reluctance to seek help because of stigma or shame associated with their condition.

Patients will probably always need the human touch in more severe cases but the digital native generation will be happy to have a video call, share their vital statistics and probably use an online service to order and manage the delivery of their prescription, and rely on automated reminders of what to take when, with background confirmation to the doctor that they took the medicine and anonymized data to the drug company of the outcome and any adverse effects.

The "PlacAppbo" Effect

Although there will continue to be much debate about the efficacy of apps, accessories, self-service diagnosis and other inventions, there is no doubt that frequently any activity that is believed to be having a positive effect on a patient may in fact bring about a comparable result to actual treatment. We may yet see the Placebo effect joined by a PlacAppbo effect when patients are treated with nothing more than an app.

Future Patients

Doctors will undoubtedly have to have a large amount of patience with a large number of patients who are over enthusiastic with new technologies. The ability to self-diagnose and self-monitor in minute detail is a boon to those with any form of hypochondriac tendencies. There will no doubt be cases where patients will will overreact and misinterpret data. But in order to prevent widespread cyberchondria, doctors will have to be in a position to encourage and educate their patients in the sensible use of devices that are relevant to them.

For their own part, doctors will have to continue to be wary of moves towards over-diagnosis as highlighted in the 2012 book *Overdiagnosed: Making People Sick in Pursuit of Health*. There is a fine line to be walked to ensure that healthcare adopts a continuous and preventative philosophy not just instead of an incident-driven and reactive system but also avoiding temptations to prematurely turn people into patients through overzealous interventions.

It seems foolish to think a patient can comprehend medical theory as well as a doctor with at least eight years studying and experience, but surely it is equally bizarre to disregard the inputs a patient can offer from their own unique position.

Finally in this topic, it's important to comment on the concept of patients rating doctors, as many apps and web sites encourage. A valuable part of e-commerce decision making and often the decisive factor for people when choosing hotels or restaurants, reviews and word of mouth are the number one factor nowadays in influencing choices in many sectors. While patients are of course entitled to their opinion and should expect courteous and professional treatment, when assessing peer reviews of doctors, you should remember that patient rating of doctors are not as straight forward as reviews of products you've bought on Amazon. Patients who don't get the prescription they want don't always rate positively and patients may have been under particular stress or vulnerability at the time of their visit.

The doctor-patient relationship as we have known it is gone. Patients will increasingly expect healthcare to be more service oriented. The consumerization of medicine and the medicalization of consumers will see changes in how and where patients see doctors, what information they provide to doctors and how patients will expect results and treatments to be delivered. For their part, doctors will face changes to decades old practices, more partially informed or even ill-informed patients as well as apps and computerized expert systems. All this against a backdrop of financial pressures and countless scientific advances in areas such as genetics and microbiota mark this as a seminal time in the history of human health.

Knowledge is Power or Ignorance is Bliss: Over-Diagnosis?

With all the emphasis and accessibility that mobile tools place on health, some people may choose to take measuring and monitoring to extremes. How much disease we find depends on how hard we look, how often we look and with what technology. Our new found powers of measurement and resultant diagnosis need to be handled with care. We need to strike a balance between promoting wellness as opposed to looking for something to be wrong. It's hard to make an asymptomatic person feel better, and reduced risk of future events is hard to quantify with any real certainty - knowing about a risk is different from being certain of an outcome.

Early detection is generally good, earlier is not necessarily better though and there are degrees of earlyness. If we do not stop to consider the appropriateness of our investigations, we could reach a point of negative return where intervening too early may label too many people as sick. A significant number of them may never have gone on to develop any meaningful symptoms; over-eager diagnosis can cause unnecessary interventions without an improvement in real outcomes. The action that people may choose to take based on an early diagnosis is not always exclusively all about the medical appropriateness - people are advised to become patients - some medical systems perversely commercially need more patients.

Not everybody wants to know their risks or potential fate or their concerns may change over time. There may be more to gain from health promotion rather than medicalizing every metric and leading to additional testing that could give unclear or incorrect pointers or cause additional anguish in cases where no effective treatment exists.

Historically, we've seen people move straight to being patients at the first sign of illness. If we can make them participants in their own health care first, we can perhaps delay the move to patients. It's an active stage rather than passive so as that suggests it requires more upfront effort. But when the time comes to be a patient, the person will be better informed and able to continue participating actively in their care.

We should soon see a future where when we get sick it is not usually a surprise. In many cases - it may be more about deciding when it makes sense to begin treatment. The diagnosis and treatment decisions would be a collaborative effort between the patient, and the doctor who will be supported by a supercomputer intelligent web service. Beyond that the next steps include decisions and treatments tailored to our own personal genomic and biomic data, all in real time.

It's important to keep this in perspective and be clear about avoiding an epidemic of cyberchondria. Whether you're measuring with mobile or traditional devices, there is of course an "appropriate" level of information. There's a temptation to over-measure looking for signs of concern just because measuring is now so easy. Just because your phone can check your vital signs anywhere anytime doesn't mean you need to or should. Unless you are feeling unwell or have been advised to by a doctor, there's little medical need to check your vital signs every day. Your weight will vary during the day every day so you can give yourself false readings if you start comparing it all the time. In most cases, a weekly routine of checking vital signs is more than observant enough.

Often originally attributed to management guru Peter Drucker, several bosses I have worked for in different industries have reminded me that "what gets measured gets managed". Applying this to your health can pay huge dividends. At the end of the day, they are tools to enable you to control and understand your health. Tools that are like DIY - better in the hands of professionals but competent when used by eager amateurs who take the time and effort to use them correctly. But we all know stories of where DIY has gone horribly wrong and professionals have had to come in and save the day. For the first time ever, the tools that are available to amateurs are a matter of life and death - we must also ensure it doesn't lead to complacency: you don't want a situation where just because a phone, sensors and apps say you're ok, you choose to ignore unusual symptoms.

Questions of Accessibility

Will this revolution of access to medical and quasi-medical information be of most benefit to a social elite? Perhaps initially it will be the better off who are most aware of and will have the most access to emerging technologies. But clearly, if affordable and pervasive technologies can democratize access to health awareness, information and medical expertise, we can look forward to a significant digital dividend.

However, in ensuring the even spread of this dividend, two groups especially come to mind when talking about access to these emerging technologies - the less well-off and the elderly. These groups have already been identified as laggards in the computer age, with access to computers and connectivity trailing badly behind other groups. Yet these are the very groups that have higher incidences of chronic health issues, coupled with the lowest ability to pay for ongoing health care.

Luckily, these groups are already embracing smartphones as prices fall and connectivity improves. Going forward, there is little cost-based rationale for these groups not to have access to some of the most recent advances. And with the affordability of devices such as activity trackers and glucometers now perhaps as low as $15 per unit, I expect government and private initiatives to focus on ensuring widespread access to these devices among vulnerable cohorts - not solely for altruistic reasons, but also in an attempt to reduce the cost of providing acute care compared to a minimal investment that may provide preventative relief. But cost is not the only factor - free isn't cheap enough to ensure people use technology. Education to create awareness and clarity about the benefits will be crucial in driving uptake.

When considering the cost of any of the devices and services in this book and considering them to be "expensive" or "affordable", I am taking the approach that most people have a smartphone anyway, and it's usually possible to spread the cost of the higher end ones over a two year contract in many cases. Even if you can't or don't want a contract to acquire a subsidized high end phone, more broadly affordable mid-range phones are well capable of handling most of the tasks described here. And if you have to prioritize your expenditure, it will be increasingly likely that you can consider a phone as a medical tool, not just a convenience.

But when it comes to whether you consider the costs of the accessories expensive, I recommend looking at them in the context of medical costs. Could they save you from expensive additional consultations or treatments? What about the time they could save you from attending clinics? Or the cost of drugs? Or, in line with the rather grand claim of the book title itself - are they expensive if they enhance or extend your life? And let's not forget the other payback - if enough people adopted a healthier lifestyle, the burden on all taxpayers could be reduced and money redirected into other services or even returned to taxpayers.

For anyone who doubts the suitability of technology-based solutions for the elderly, I would point to the increasing number of silver surfers who prove willing to consider new technologies if they are clearly beneficial and made accessible to older age groups. As the technology rapidly becomes more user friendly (take the app that just looks at you to track your heart rate for example), coupled with the instinctive reliance on technology of their supporting younger generations, we will see mobile technology increasingly employed to benefit the elderly. It would be a shame if those potentially most in line to benefit miss out from a lack of awareness or access. And longer term, the economics of proactively providing them with such access may far outweigh the cost, both human and financial, of not taking measures to ensure nobody is left out.

As the world's population ages rapidly, solutions focused on improving the quality of life for the ageing will undoubtedly proliferate. From the continuous monitoring of vital signs, compliance with prescriptions and monitoring of falls to the availability of on-demand remote video consultations, there is every chance that old age will become better cared for than ever before. Independent living can be sustained more safely than in the past, and residential care can be improved too - if you have an elderly relative in a care home and are worried about the level of attention they are receiving, why not slip an activity tracking watch on them - next time you visit you'll be able to tell if they are getting the daily exercise the care home claims.

Health at Home

A hospital is no place to be sick

- Samuel Goldwyn

The rise of remote consultations and app-based prescription ordering for delivery will see people make fewer visits to doctor's offices and clinics, as well as potentially leading to a drop in hospital attendance. Remote monitoring may see increasing numbers of people cared for at home. A move away from hospital-centered care may seem counter-intuitive in terms of improved outcomes but if managed carefully, it may bring big benefits, both financial and in reducing infection risk. Care at home, where practical, can reduce the risk of the infections encountered in such institutions despite their best efforts at hygiene regimes - nosocomial (originating in a hospital) and iatrogenic (caused by doctor or treatment) infections, which combine to kill thousands of hospital patients each year.

Across the Globe

Most of the discussion in this book to date has been around the emergence of mobile-enhanced medical opportunities that depend on modern smartphones and high speed cellular or broadband connectivity. I've also focused on how these technologies can help us tackle health issues that are widely seen in the developed world.

But these and related technological advances will have differing impacts in different parts of the world. While the developed world increasingly faces so-called 21st century diseases having largely banished pathogenic infectious diseases, there are still many parts of the world where healthcare has a different focus. In the US, the deaths caused by communicable diseases stands at 6%, whereas it stands at over 70% in many African countries.

In several cases, developing countries already have a greater reliance on 2G mobile technologies such as SMS notifications, for patient education and reminders, compared to many industrialized nations where other channels and media exist. Frequently, developing countries have much greater mobile infrastructure than healthcare delivery coverage. Just as many of these countries have skipped an entire generation of technology such as fixed phone lines, they now stand to skip a generation of centralized medical services which are limited by proximity. The role that mobile technology plays may vary in different countries - it is important to remember that although they have rapidly growing and connected populations, not all are the same in terms of smartphone ownership or underlying health care challenges, access to drugs or payment models. But as the cost of smartphones continues to tumble, and access to connectivity improves rapidly via initiatives such as those being trialed already by Google and Facebook for balloon and drone-based internet access, there must be real hope that dramatic improvements in health in recent years in the developing world can be sustained or even accelerated.

Institutional Impacts

According to PwC, Mobile health services can be categorized into two broad areas: solutions across the "Patient Pathway" and "Healthcare Systems Strengthening". The Patient Pathway - Wellness, Prevention, Diagnosis, Treatment and Monitoring - entail direct touch-points with patients and with the advent of mobile technologies, are rapidly being devolved to the patient themselves. Healthcare Systems Strengthening solutions refer to the clinical, hospital or administration systems that frequently do not involve direct interactions with patients, but are primarily aimed at improving the efficiency of healthcare providers in delivering patient care.

In this book, we're mainly concerned with the patient-level technologies - the advances that you can have access to at minimal cost, often in the palm of your hand. Yet these don't exist in isolation - harnessing these to their fullest will be driven by and drive changes in institutional systems too. Consumer mobile health must be considered in tandem with hospital systems such as Electronic Health Records (EHR), the IT operational mainstay of a modern hospital. EHRs do not yet have a good reputation among the medical community but these short-term challenges will be overcome as technology, processes and users mature. For anyone looking to understand the opportunities and challenges around these large healthcare systems deployment, I recommend "The Digital Doctor: Hope, Hype, and Harm at the Dawn of Medicine's Computer" by Robert Wachter.

The 2015 annual HealthCare's Most Wired survey by the American Hospital Association's Health Forum and the College of Healthcare Information Management Executives (CHIME) shows that Health data security and patient engagement are top priorities for US hospitals. Among their key findings were that 89 percent of Most Wired organizations offer access to the patient portal through a mobile application, 67 percent of Most Wired hospitals already offer the ability to incorporate patient-generated data and 63 percent offer self-management tools for chronic conditions.

Just as consumers and doctors will take advantage of falling prices and increasing capabilities of sensor technologies and mobile devices, hospitals will also see a massive upheaval in the coming years with mobile-based technologies permeating the corridors and specialties of hospitals with an array of dedicated solutions complying with the onerous privacy and encryption regime imposed on hospitals by legislation such as HIPAA which require that apps ensure no identifiable patient information falls into unapproved hands. Examples include secure peer to peer messaging systems such as MedXnote (like What's App Messenger but secured for Doctors) and even an app from Gauss Surgical that estimates how much blood a sponge or swab has absorbed just by taking a photo off it - useful for surgeons trying to estimate blood loss in a patient.

Embracing change will require support at the highest levels in healthcare administration. In an interview with the Guardian in January 2015, NHS England's Medical director outlined his views that mobile technology would play a key role in the future of the service. Prof. Sir Bruce Keogh pointed to devices which not only measure how much exercise you do but can also measure your heart rate, your respiratory rate, and whether or not you've got excess fluid in your body – quite complex changes in your physiology - which health professionals can analyze and then act upon any warning signs.

"I see a time where someone who's got heart failure because they've had a previous heart attack is sitting at home and wearing some unobtrusive sensors, and his phone goes, and it's a health professional saying: 'Mr Smith, we've been monitoring you and we think you're starting to go back into heart failure. Someone's going to be with you in half an hour to give you some diuretics'," says Keogh. Technology "enables you to predict things, to act early and to prevent unnecessary admissions, thereby not only taking a load off the NHS but, more importantly, actually keeping somebody safe and feeling good". Over the next few years the NHS will push forward with "a huge rollout" of such devices as part of "a revolution in self-care".

Further figures from the NHS reveal that 97% of GPs now offer online appointments, repeat prescriptions and access to summary information in medical records, benefitting more than 55 million patients across England. This is up from 3% just over a year ago. The NHS believes that giving people the opportunity to cancel and rebook appointments online will help to reduce the number of missed appointments, currently estimated to cost around £160 million ($250m) per year.

Chapter 11:
Data & The Big Picture

Man will become better when you show him what he's like.

- Anton Chekhov

More data has been generated in the 18 months since I started writing this book than in the entire history of mankind before that time. This is truly information overload on a mind-boggling scale. But while we generate information at an astonishing rate, thankfully we are also getting much better at analyzing that data and finding the meanings hidden within it. History will doubtless recognize the smartphone and its associated technologies as the most significant advance in communications and data since the printing press, and one that will likely grow to dwarf the significance of even that defining event in the generation, preservation and dissemination of information.

Scanadu, the maker of the tricorder-like vital signs sensor I described in Chapter 3, promote its strap line as "we're the last generation to know so little about our health" and I believe that is absolutely correct. Simply wearing a single activity tracker generates literally thousands of data points per hour. If you decide to monitor vital signs too you, are soon into the tens of thousands for just an individual's routine on-going measurements.

Reade Harpham, the director of human-centric design at Battelle Memorial Institute, points out that a couple of years ago, developers and researchers might get 200 data points a day about parameters such as somebody's diet, exercise, glucose levels, heartbeat, and how he or she reacts to certain treatments. Now some pharmaceutical companies are tackling 18 million data points, per patient, per day, about genetics, reactions to drugs, and environmental stimuli, Harpham says. So as we uncover ever more data about the human condition, the more important question is whether, when faced with facts and insights, we're the last generation to do so little about improving our health.

Having huge amounts of information is a double-edged sword. Buried within the data are undoubtedly insights, trends and clues, surrogate outcomes you can manipulate towards the outcomes you want. But the data also obscure findings, introduce paranoia and raise privacy, regulatory and policy questions. While this may seem daunting to many, a parallel technology to the miniaturization of sensors is the explosion of technology to interpret all this data. Algorithms embedded in smartphone apps can analyze the data that you generate - or dispatch the data to be remotely processed via cloud computing.

Processing large quantities of data is what computers are good at - as part of their research on enabling health care improvements via technology, IBM says each person generates one million gigabytes of health-related data across his or her lifetime, the equivalent of more than 300 million average sized books. The IBM "Watson" supercomputer can read the equivalent of a million books a second so data size isn't the challenge...it's making it useful and IBM recently created a dedicated business unit to figure out how Watson's immense computation powers can be augmented to pull out individualized insights to help people and providers make timely, evidence-based decisions about health-related issues.

If we get so-called "Big Data" right in healthcare, the benefits should be enormous: The McKinsey Global Institute estimates that applying big-data strategies to better inform decision making could generate up to $100 billion in value annually across the US health-care system, by optimizing innovation, improving the efficiency of research and clinical trials, and building new tools for physicians, consumers, insurers and regulators to deliver on the promise of more individualized approaches.

For me, there are three main questions with all this new-found data and access to metrics on virtually everything you do.....how is it useful or actionable, to whom is it useful and who is in control of it all? Let's look at how it can be made useful at an individual level, before moving on to the other levels to consider - corporate and public health.

Bringing It All Together For An Individual

All of the apps mentioned here collect vast amounts of data. Most do a good job at shielding you from the raw data and analyzing it. You can take a proactive approach and go into the app(s) each day to get a summary of how you are doing, or most also offer a weekly email summary if you want to take a more hands-off approach. Be ready though for the fact that most apps try hard to keep you engaged, with frequent notifications popping up to ask you for more information (in the case of food tracking, that's around every meal time) or to keep you motivated (it's 8pm and you've only got 2,000 steps - not much time left today!).

However, the disjointed nature of most apps which only focus on one or two areas means it's still difficult to get an overall view. Many apps allow you to exchange data via Application Programming Interfaces - APIs - three crucial letters in the internet age that most people aren't aware of but which enable the flow of information between different systems at an unprecedented rate. But even though my Withings weighing scales can tell my Jawbone activity tracker what my weight is, and the so-called Smartcoach in the Jawbone Up app will then try to analyze all the information to find correlations between for example weight loss and activity or sleep levels, it's still not a complete picture. Google, Apple, Microsoft and Samsung have each tried to create central repositories of health information to connect multiple sources in an attempt to build a more comprehensive picture from disparate sources.

Although we talked about activity trackers in Chapter 4 and their focus on steps, the actual amount of data collected is mind-boggling. For each "step" you take, multiple data points are recorded - the movement itself, but also the force of the movement, the movement of your hips, the number of movements per minute, the location of the movement - so at the simplest level, that's 120 data points per minute. Sleep sensors record your movement, breaths, heartbeats, snores - all continuously as you sleep. This level of detail is, of course, of no interest to most people and in order for mobile technologies to deliver on their promise, it is vital that people shouldn't have to worry about this minutia, get bogged down in the details, nor battle multiple apps unless they are after a very specific view.

Aggregation & Analysis

Enter aggregation and analysis services shared by multiple apps using API technologies invisible to users - the wisdom being that the combined information can be made more valuable that the individual parts - where the data is turned into actionable information. There are now many apps and services which try to make sense of all the disparate sources of data, looking for relationships, insights and causes. In a slightly strange journey, much of the information that originates from sensors within the phone, is sent to services in the cloud, only to return to the phone's screen in summary form, hopefully with some added value. So what sort of information do these provide?

- Services like zenobase.com provide a dashboard that answers simple questions - e.g. what impact does room temperature have on your sleep - by combining data from your Netatmo Environment sensor with your Jawbone sleep data.

- Addapp allows you to connect any of 35 different services and it will offer personalized insights by cross-referencing, for example, your sleep data and your activity data - it can make explicit connections you probably already could guess - like the days you sleep less than average you are more likely to take the elevator instead of the stairs. While most of its connections are in the activity and food tracking spaces, interestingly it is able to include your Uber usage and your location check-ins so can add value to your health information by referencing your transport and location information. While insights such as getting a cab instead of walking provides less steps might be obvious, the potential to discover how you gain weight the days you go certain places (fast food restaurants) or don't go to other places (gym) may surface a few startling choices for you to make.

- One approach to make all the health data more understandable is provided by a service called Dacadoo. This combines the data feeds from apps, watches, trackers, scales and cardiac monitors to create a combined health score. This single number from 1 to 1,000 is based on a variety of inputs including nutrition; exercise; emotional wellbeing; lifestyle choices; sleep patterns and stress. This holistic balanced-scorecard style approach has the benefit of ensuring that you don't focus solely on one aspect of your overall well-being. As only a certain proportion of your health score is determined by exercise, hitting your steps target every day at the expense of healthy eating or regular sleeping or management of stress will not increase your overall health score. Tracking over time with a simple number allows you to see trends and then drill down into what's causing a drop in your score.

- Tictrac is another aggregation and analysis service, but takes a different approach. Rather than trying to find correlations or simplify things into a health score, it offers anyone interested enough a means to analyze their own information to find patterns themselves. As with the other services, it relies on your granting permission to access the data feeds from your activity trackers, but expands much further to include entertainment (books read, music listened to) and social activity (Facebook, Twitter). This drag and drop tool lets you overlay (or "slice and dice" in analytics parlance) your activities by time of day and, for anyone who takes the time, it can reveal lifestyle interactions you would never normally notice. Predefined templates make it easy to get started with suggested services to link, but be prepared to visualize your life in ways you never imagined - did you know you tend to post on Twitter and Instagram more on the days you eat particular foods? And while maybe you secretly know you watch a bit too much TV, it's quite stark to see it graphed for you over a year, and even more impactful to see your activity levels overlaid with it and your weight on the same graph.

- Alternatively, if you are keen to be involved in research rather than a commercial system, you can join in with Intel's data visualization experiment at makesenseofdata.com. This is a research experiment designed by a group of anthropologists, designers and computer scientists at Intel Labs, in collaboration with Savage Internet and Empiricala to explore whether it is possible to build tools to improve data literacy without making people into statisticians. They point to an example of one researcher who was tracking the healthiness level of her food. Using a type of analysis similar to a "periodic pattern" tool, she discovered that her food healthiness dips on Mondays and Wednesdays – exactly when her partner works late into the evening, and they go out to eat together.

- For anyone who wants to explore their data in even more detail, then consider the organization Quantifiedself.com where you can attend a meetup of like-minded individuals, or consider creating your own visualization with the open source tool https://fluxtream.org/.

- One interesting specialist platform that is aiming to take the information from phones, analyze it and link to medical providers is Ginger.io. Their system uses MIT-developed machine learning and data mining to passively collect and analyze subtle signals of behavior change to better understand users' social, physical and mental health status. By monitoring your mood, interactions with other people and movements, this app intends to identify any concerning changes in behavior patterns, or a lack of response, and alert your caregivers. Their stated aim is to drive better behavioral health outcomes through the use of passive mobile data and behavioral analytics to support patients with depression, anxiety disorders, schizophrenia, and bipolar disorder.

- It can be daunting for smaller healthcare technology providers looking to interact with so many data sources and there are now broker services emerging that are designed to create a one-to-many connection to digital health technologies. HumanAPI and Validic are examples of cloud-based platforms that connect patient-recorded data from digital health apps and accessories to other healthcare stakeholders like hospital systems, insurers and health consultants. Again using API technology, developers of health systems can treat these systems as a "black box" that gives them access to all the various data gathering platforms out there (over 175 at the time of writing in the case of Validic) without having to know the details of each one. This kinds of services open possibilities for smaller innovators and entrepreneurs to connect with, and attempt to add value to, a virtually endless stream of data.

If all this sounds a bit Orwellian, then remember that you are in control of what information and services you link. Vinod Khosla, a co-founder of 1990s computer giant Sun Microsystems and prolific investor in mobile health start-ups, said recently "As we have more and more sophisticated wearables that can continuously measure things ranging from your physical activity to your stress levels to your emotional state, we can begin to cross-correlate and understand how each aspect of our life consciously and unconsciously impacts one another". But there remain interesting conundrums about other parties that might stand to benefit from your data; with whom and exactly what you decide to share will become a more pressing issue.

Health Technology in the Workplace

If your boss asks you how you are, you may wonder that's out of genuine concern or, more likely, a worry that you might be sick and about to cost sick pay and/or a loss of productivity. Nowadays though, the question may have been prompted because they've been alerted that your heart rate has been higher than usual for the last few days, a fact available to them as mobile health technologies are increasingly deployed in the workplace.

It's long been commonplace to undergo a medical exam as part of most job application processes. Usually fairly superficial in nature, this is often the first and final medical involvement for employers, other than processing occasional sick notes. More recently, it has become reasonably common practice for more conscientious employers to provide some form of corporate wellness program - which can range from subsidized gym memberships to screening sessions to free fruit snacks in offices. But now, some employers are starting to take an interest in employee well-being beyond these simple gestures and venturing into territory that raises significant legal and ethical questions.

Your work has a clear connection to your well-being. A recent survey by Withings, quoted in Forbes, revealed that most people gain weight when they start a new job. Most people spend a huge proportion of their lives in work and in most cases, the workplace is a safe place, even in industries which have historically been injurious to health. Many people are familiar with health and safety training but, in my experience, it focuses on the safety aspect far more - and while accident avoidance is laudable, the promotion of health is usually overlooked once employees have watched the safe lifting video. And while companies have a duty of care under legislation to protect workers from harm, where do you draw the line? Do companies have a responsibility to protect you from your own less-than-ideal lifestyle habits that will end up costing them money even if you don't care about them potentially costing you your life? What about a responsibility to protect you from subtle dangers like requiring you to sit for extended periods, even in your very expensive lumbar-supporting chair?

Given the challenges people face in finding time to dedicate to their well-being, having it provided/supported/mandated by their employer can, at least partially, remove that particular barrier. Employers may find that it increases pressure on them too - while they could pay lip service to wellness programs such as paying for your gym membership with no attendance follow-up, it will become clear if workloads are precluding people from taking their recommended level of steps, and staff may be able to use that against companies who fail to provide time or access to health facilities.

Which Technologies?

The mobile technologies that have moved into the consumer mainstream are also now visible in the corporate space, alongside services that are specifically aimed at the business market. It remains to be seen how appropriate these devices are in the workplace and which of the nearly endless metrics that can be counted should be counted and shared in a professional setting.

The emergence of affordable solutions gives a new impetus to the area of corporate wellness and existing fitness tracker providers:

- Withings http://corporate.withings.com/
- Jawbone http://groups.jawbone.com
- Fitbit http://www.fitbit.com/fitbit-wellness

who have adapted their services to create offerings for use in a corporate setting - allowing companies to create closed user groups where different departments can compete against each other to complete the most steps in a given time period. Some employers provide the tracking devices free of charge, hopeful that the investment will be easily repaid by any reduction in sick days from their more health conscious staff. At the level of daily steps information, I see little reason not to share my steps with colleagues. But do I want them to know that I didn't get much sleep last night? Or as trackers get more advanced and record vital signs such as heart rate, do I want to risk that information being made available to my colleagues?

Dedicated providers like https://omadahealth.com/ offer tailored schemes with live coaches supported by apps. Dacadoo, mentioned earlier, also offers a version of its health score platform adapted for corporate use.

There have been a number of studies about the impact of these technologies in the workplace. One example, The Human Cloud At Work study led by Dr Chris Brauer of the Institute of Management Studies at Goldsmiths, University of London found that productivity for people using wearable technology increased 8.5 per cent. However, it's still early to form a long term picture, so you have to be very wary of the "Hawthorne Effect", a psychology term coined to highlight the fact that employees are apt to change their behavior just because they are being studied.

Companies can feel a significant financial burden of an unhealthy workforce with increased absenteeism, disability, injury and rising healthcare costs. The Centers for Disease Control and Prevention (CDC) has shown that companies with workplace wellness programs can yield a 3x return for each dollar invested in such programs. Corporate Wellness is not a new concept but the existing web-based platforms based on health assessments, coupled with educational content, tips and eventually online videos, fail to create the sort of engagement that mobile technology can achieve so the next time the CDC runs their research, the results may be even better.

The Partnership for Prevention and US Chamber of Commerce published a document in 2001 entitled Healthy Workforce 2010 targeting 75% of US organizations, large and small, to enact a corporate wellness initiative. In health, new rules under The Affordable Care Act (Obamacare) broaden the incentives employers can give their staff, boosting cash rewards on premiums or deductibles from 20% to 30%. Small businesses can apply to a pot of $200 million in grants to set up such programs.

The cynical will perceive that most workplace wellness programs are probably motivated more by concerns over lost productivity or rising healthcare costs (especially in the US where employer funded medical care is a bigger concern than other countries where employers are historically less involved in funding) than any sense of duty towards employees. But regardless of the motivation, if the outcome is better for the individual in terms of education about lifestyle changes, provision of healthier food or subsidized access to assistive technologies, then I can excuse the underlying rationale. However, questions will inevitably be raised regarding issues such as employees being required to participate and intrusion across the work/life divide. And while team bonding or friendly inter-departmental rivalries are to be encouraged, will leaderboards add to office camaraderie or provoke unhelpful rivalries? While I've already highlighted the proven benefits of support from friends or contacts within wellness apps, it's far from certain that extending that to the workplace will deliver the same beneficial results in a work setting.

Of course workplace wellness is not just about steps or what you eat or providing bicycle parking racks. It can also extend to stress management. With some 70% of US workers said to be suffering from work-related stress, there is an argument that employers have a duty to provide their staff with the knowhow and tools to better manage this. But this move beyond the physical is venturing into very personal territory. It also raises questions about those taking sick days where the medical grounds for such an absence may not entirely stack up. If your wearable monitor reports that your temperature is fine, you'd better not call in and claim a "fever".

Informed Consent

A 2015 survey from PwC claims that more than half of employees would consider wearing a smartwatch from their employer if their data were used to improve things such as working hours, stress levels and where they can work from. PwC's research with over 2,000 working UK adults reveals that trust is the main barrier to people being willing to share their personal data with their employer - two fifths (41%) said they don't trust their employer not to use the data against them in some way and a similar amount (40%) said they don't trust their employer to use the data for their benefit. Lawyers say companies would have to gain the explicit informed consent of employees before gathering personal data from wearables — and further consent to correlate it with other data, such as performance metrics.

While I believe that people struggling to find the time or motivation to embrace healthier lifestyles may be greatly assisted by corporate supports for their endeavors, this is a sensitive issue and needs to be managed with care by HR policy makers. To get a more in-depth sense of the issues raised, you might find it interesting to read a special report by the Financial Times in May 2015 which elicited, and duly provoked, strong feedback - https://www.facebook.com/wearablesatwork.

The Health of Nations

While I've concentrated thus far primarily on the individual impact of mobile technologies, given that both mobile phones and your health are very personal considerations, it is worth noting that the advances made possible in this arena may have significant implications for public health, if policy makers and health administrators embrace the changes. The focus of the book is on the technology available to the individual to improve their well-being. But to place it in proper context, we must examine the bigger picture of health care challenges at a national and even international scale. Many of the personal gains within our grasp could be multiplied hugely at a macro scale.

If mobile technologies can deliver improvements at an individual level in preventative lifestyle changes, chronic disease management and drug adherence, these sum to massive national returns. But many social scientists are now imagining a future where parallel developments and deployments of sensors at an urban level will combine with our health data to create smarter cities.

Buried in the aggregate data being gathered by millions of affordable personal sensor devices are patterns that may reveal what factors in the diet, exercise regimen and environment contributes to disease. These cheap devices will keep track of your own health but they can also be easily used to detect infection outbreaks at a national or pandemic level, with people anonymously uploading data to a cloud. The Centers for Disease Control or the World Health Organization could quite literally keep their fingers on the pulse of the entire planet. More locally and less dramatically, patterns could be used to help inform urban planners and healthcare planners where facilities are needed or district education campaigns might be effective.

Beyond Curiosity

The validity and usefulness of much of the data currently being collected by the various apps, trackers and sensors is still unclear to many people. Until the use of these technologies becomes more widespread, and extends beyond its current heartland of worried well and begins the reach a statistically representative level, you have to remember that we don't yet have a reliable snapshot of the health of the nation. But already we can start to see signs of the kinds of information that will be available once we remove the self-selection bias of people with an active interest in monitoring their well-being.

One of the leading providers of smart health technology, Withings (who make scales, activity trackers and blood pressure monitors mentioned earlier) have made anonymized data from their users available via a dedicated web site (http://obs.withings.com/) - this gives you State-level data you can interrogate to understand levels of obesity and high blood pressure sourced directly from individuals. For example, according to the analysis of over 100,000 Withings users, Mississippi is the least active state in the US, with DC being the most. Over in Europe, Iceland has the highest overweight rate, while Latvia has the lowest.

Epidemics?

While we've talked mainly about your own health and what's within your control, and as we've noted most infectious diseases have been largely controlled in the industrialized world, there are of course many illnesses that are communicable, some serious and some no more menacing than the common cold.

There are now several Illness tracking apps such as SickWeather and HealthyDay that search social media for keywords or enable users to post their status and create a crowd-sourced map of illnesses, allowing you to see a visual representation of who has a series of common ailments on your street—from garden-variety colds to the flu and chicken pox. This kind of data might be useful in identifying the spread of illness for local health authorities, or if you are in a vulnerable cohort, you could avoid areas of known high infection rates during flu season. The CDC have their own app called FluView. This allows users to monitor levels of influenza across the country, including views of Influenza Like Illness (ILI) trends over several weeks. FluView gathers its data from more than 3,000 health care providers in all 50 states, the District of Columbia, and the U.S. Virgin Islands, reporting more than 30 million patient visits each year.

While the exponential growth of social networks demonstrates our desire to share and our frequent inability to filter what we share, things may change when it comes to health data. As long as my blood pressure is ok, then I have no hesitation in sharing it. But if it is somewhat less than ideal, then sharing it may be ill-advised. Will my boss take it into consideration when choosing the next promotion candidates? Will my life assurer and my health insurer take it into account? If my neighborhood shows high illness rates on one of the apps above, might that adversely affect property values?

Regulation

The changes being wrought by the availability of new technologies focused on health and well-being, the addition of vast quantities of new products, new services and new entrants are together disrupting the landscape that has existed in relative calm for many years. As regular consumers, medical professionals, data analysts and corporations grapple with if, how and when to best embrace change, the regulatory framework is facing unprecedented upheaval.

Medicine has always been a highly regulated profession, to ensure as far as possible quality of care for patients. The College of Physicians was founded in 1518 and competed with the Church for licensing physicians. Modern regulation began in 1858 with the establishment of what is now known as the General Medical Council in the UK. More recent bodies such as The new National Institute for Clinical Excellence, National Patient Safety Agency and Council for Healthcare Regulatory Excellence (CHRE) have enhanced control over medical quality, professional decision making and surveillance of care provider performance. Over the years, different countries have taken different approaches to regulation and there are now multiple specialist regulatory authorities in most jurisdictions complicating matters further. The European Commission does much to coordinate medical regulation across the EU, while the Food and Drug Administration (FDA) is responsible for the regulation of medical devices in the US with the Federal Trace Commission (FTC) responsible for apps.

Although often criticized, it should be acknowledged that regulators face a difficult task: first and foremost, they must keep people safe and apply reasonable precautions to ensure appropriate education and competence amongst those licensed to practice and supply healthcare devices and services. But they must also look for ways to leverage new technologies for good, encourage innovation and somehow avoid stifling progress. All of this within an environment where costs must be tightly controlled and in the face of device manufacturers pushing to release new technologies, patient groups telling harrowing stories in an effort to get experimental drugs accelerated and, increasingly, individuals who believe they have the right to determine their own treatments, even if based on information from apps that have no medical validity.

Regulating Accessories

If you consider that just a couple of years ago, much of the technology I am discussing either didn't exist or wasn't affordably accessible, it's not surprising that the innovation is outpacing the scientific and legal framework for testing and regulating such devices. In an effort to keep up the Food and Drug Administration in January 2015 proposed an updated stance which indicated it would continue to comprehensively regulate devices that are invasive, but take a lighter touch on other offerings, creating a policy for low risk products that just promote a healthy lifestyle or what it termed "general wellness products".
According to the FDA, these general wellness products are defined as products that meet the following two factors: (1) they are intended for only general wellness use, and (2) they present a very low risk to users' safety.

However, the FDA want to make clear that a product's inclusion under this guidance does not establish that it has been shown to be safe, effective, and not misbranded for its intended use. According to the agency's draft guidelines, a wellness product crosses into the territory of a medical device (which requires a rigorous FDA review that is time consuming and expensive for manufacturers) when its intended use refers to a specific disease or condition, or it presents an inherent risk to a user's safety.

Such general wellness products would still be subject to monitoring by the Consumer Product Safety Commission, which has the power to recall products to protect the public against unreasonable risks from injuries or death from consumer products. In 2014, after some users complained of skin irritations from Fitbit Force activity tracking bands, the CPSC worked with the company on a recall that affected more than 1 million devices.

Regulating Apps

When it comes to the ever-expanding world of apps, the regulatory environment is far from clear. Consider a situation where an unscrupulous app developer makes available an app that claims to scan a photo that a user uploads and determine if they have a particular condition, e.g. melanoma. Trouble is the developer has no medical skills, has not developed an amazing algorithm that can detect cancer more effectively than a human expert and has instead just set a random generator to review the photo but charges $10 to "review" each photo...Who is responsible for oversight in this kind of scenario?

With new apps being uploaded at the rate of over 500 per day, the regulator can hardly find and review every single app that makes any form of medical claim. To do so, they would need unmanageable amounts of staff to review them. Is it Google/Apple's responsibility as the owner of the app stores? Hardly, as they are not qualified to judge if the app is performing a medical function as claimed. Both Google and Apple have comprehensive Terms of Service for their app stores and reserve the right to remove any apps found to be in breach of these terms. A link enabling users to report concerns about the quality of any app is readily available in the app stores.

A recent case take by the FTC provides a good example: the action against two melanoma detection apps which claimed to provide an "automated analysis of moles and skin lesions for symptoms of melanoma and increase consumers' chances of detecting melanoma in its early stages" led to settlements of just over of $20,000.

But, interestingly, there was disagreement within the FTC on the case - one FTC Commissioner Maureen Ohlhausen agreed that apps must have substantial scientific backing in order to make claims, but she questioned just how high that bar should be. "This approach concerns me," she wrote. "Health-related apps have enormous potential to improve access to health information for underserved populations and to enable individuals to monitor more effectively their own well-being, thereby improving health outcomes. Health-related apps need not be as accurate as professional care to provide significant value for many consumers. The [FTC] should not subject such apps to overly stringent substantiation requirements, so long as developers adequately convey the limitations of their products. In particular, the [FTC] should be very wary of concluding that consumers interpret marketing for health-related apps as claiming that those apps substitute for professional medical care, unless we can point to express claims, clearly implied claims, or extrinsic evidence. If the Commission continues to adopt such conclusions without any evidence of consumers' actual interpretations, and thus requires a very high level of substantiation for health-related apps, we are likely to chill innovation in such apps, limit the potential benefits of this innovation, and ultimately make consumers worse off."

The NHS in the UK has tackled the issue of app safety by creating a website that reviews apps against published criteria - All apps submitted to the Health Apps Library are checked to make sure that they are relevant to people living in England; comply with data protection laws and comply with trusted sources of information, such as NHS Choices which is the UK's biggest health website. Users can report any app they have concerns about and the NHS engages with the developers as necessary. But while the NHS is keen to strike a balance between promoting the use of apps and patient safety, there is a pragmatic approach from the NHS Clinical Director for Patient Safety (Dr Maureen Baker): *"Of course, we can never assure anything to be 100% safe. Crossing the road is not 100% safe but if you stop, look and listen, you are much less likely to come to harm. That's what we are trying to achieve with the Health Apps Library Review Process."*

Dr. David Bates, the chief innovation officer and senior vice president at Partners' Brigham and Women's Hospital in Boston, has conducted research into the state of medical apps. His approach included a literature review, interviews with experts, a review of apps in the App Store, and a usability study. He and his team identified a few hundred apps that targeted high-need, high-cost patients. Most of the reviewed apps' primary purpose was the display or recording of patient information, but only a few included reminders or alerts, guided the patient, or provided educational information. In addition, only 11 percent of the apps identified included both clinical experts and patients in their development process and only 22 percent rewarded the user in any way for achieving health goals. More concerning, Bates said, was the fact that only 33 percent of apps appropriately warned users in potentially dangerous situations.

"Our takeaways were that although apps have the potential to improve healthcare, they also have the potential to cause harm as they become increasingly integrated with the healthcare system," he said. "And we did identify some cases in which, for example, patients could enter a very low blood glucose level and they did not get any notification that that was important. In other apps you could tell the app that you were suicidal and it wasn't clear that anyone would be alerted."

It is ultimately probably going to be a mixture of formal and informal checks and balances and it will take a while before any sustainable regulation emerges. Just like any new wild frontier, there will be winners and losers, and some casualties along the way. Hopefully the number of app developers preying on the vulnerable or paranoid will be small. The threat of legal action from making false claims may be sufficient deterrent in most cases, with community reviews exposing fraudsters quickly. I have no doubt that further regulatory schemes will emerge and app quality will improve. Reviews and ratings will weed out the worst and patient groups as well as regulators will challenge apps that pose a risk to users. Expert recommendations for useful apps will perhaps become more important in the field of medical/well-being apps than for any other category.

So regulators are undoubtedly in a tough spot - they are in the unenviable position of being accused of luddite-ism and stifling bureaucracy, until such time as one smartphone user mis-diagnoses themselves and threatens to sue the authorities for not protecting them from themselves. At the end of the day a degree of common sense must prevail - users must be educated to treat the smartphone as an assistant or a second opinion - not the sole and immediate decision maker. In fairness, virtually all of the health and well-being apps I have seen come with very clear warnings to users that they are not medical in grade and advise users to consult a trained professional.

Data Concerns

Some physicians, academics and ethicists criticize the utility of activity tracking as prime evidence of the narcissism of the modern technological age. Des Spence, a UK GP, wrote a cautionary piece in the April 2015 issue of BMJ, the former British Medical Journal, arguing that unnecessary monitoring is creating in-cred-ible anxiety among today's "unhealthily health-obsessed" trackers. "Health and fitness have become the new social currency, spawning a 'worried well' generation". The trend also raises serious questions about the accuracy and privacy of the health data collected, who owns it and how it should be used.

Data Privacy

Concern about the quality of apps is not only about whether or not the apps are fit for purpose (however you define that) but an added layer of complexity is the worry over the security of the data generated by the various mobile technologies now flooding the market.

How the data generated from the devices is protected and shared is not always clear. Federal patient privacy rules under the Health Insurance Portability and Accountability Act (HIPAA) don't apply to most of the information these new gadgets are tracking. Unless the data is being used by a physician to treat a patient, the companies that help track a person's information aren't bound by the same confidentiality, notification and security requirements as the professional systems used in a clinic or hospital.

To make matters worse, privacy isn't a static concept. Information you may be happy to share today (my blood pressure is fine) may change to information you are far more worried about sharing (my blood pressure is now indicative of hypertension), especially if you've chosen to share it previously with your employer.

Your health data is undoubtedly precious and it's important to take reasonable steps to protect it - use safe passwords, use only reputable sites, etc. But let's face it, a security/privacy breach will likely happen at some point. I console myself that someone could break into my doctor's office and steal my file and I never worried about that. That is not to absolve those holding my data of their utmost efforts to protect my data, but I have to remain realistic that it may one day be compromised.

Outlook

More information does not always equal better. It will likely take time for norms to emerge and there may be interim periods of over-reaction, doctors being inundated with patients self-diagnosing with all manner of exotic and unlikely ailments. But just as this happened with the first access to online tools like WebMD, eventually the field normalized and people started to gravitate towards trustworthy sites while medical professionals began to see the benefits of broader information availability. In time too, I believe people, and the apps that track them, will mature to focus on compelling, insightful and actionable data.

Chapter 12: Conclusions

The previous 11 chapters have hopefully managed to give you a useful description of the radical enablers, changes, possibilities and challenges facing us and our well-being in the coming years. The advent of the smartphone phone represents the biggest change agent in well-being and health care since the arrival and widespread adoption of antibiotics or x-rays. These two momentous advances have saved millions of lives and dramatically changed public health and health practices in recent decades but they have not come without consequences. In the case of antibiotics especially, their suspected impact on the emergence of non-infectious diseases is now a priority area for further scientific investigation. So too as mobile and related technologies take root, we need to be on the lookout for consequences and impacts alongside their positive force for progress. Many of the questions that these technologies will pose are not easy or palatable for some individuals or even at a societal level.

When new technologies are becoming available at the rate they are, it's hard to measure the pace of change and even harder to measure the pace of progress - and vital that the two aren't confused as the same thing. It's worth pausing to consider the implications, both positive and negative, of widespread adoption of mobile technology as a pillar of future health policy. We cannot expect that it will all magically fall into place to create a utopian healthy society for everybody. Far from making life easier for people, emerging technologies place much greater emphasis on personal involvement in well-being than ever before. But the potential dividend for individuals and society of a longer or healthier life seems hard to ignore.

It's Early Days

When thinking about the potential applications of mobile technology to health and well-being it is important to remember that this is a young and rapidly evolving area. Neither the medical profession nor the policy makers have caught up with it, let alone assumed a position of leadership.

To put things in context, for medical practices we've had two thousand years of medical practice no more sophisticated than blood-letting, which gave way to two hundred years of science-based treatments and now perhaps we've had not much more than two years of focus on mobile medicine. The products available already will soon seem old-fashioned and will have been replaced by sleeker devices that are cheaper, more accurate, easier to use and less obtrusive. This category of technology will evolve rapidly. This year's leading devices will soon look ridiculously old fashioned and incapable. But it's not about the devices. It's about the focus they allow, the conversations they facilitate and the choices they enable. It's not too soon to get involved - today's offerings are more than good enough to help you embrace a healthier lifestyle. Not everything we've been talking about is even new - in many cases, the technology being applied is just taking proven sensible things like monitoring weight and automating it - "removing friction" to use a favored Silicon Valley term.

As with many revolutionary technologies, an important factor here is the extension of information and capabilities to new groups of people previously denied them. While I wouldn't recommend using these types of products without first seeking the advice of a medical professional, those unable to, or not inclined to, frequent doctors' surgeries may benefit from greater access to home monitoring and access to information they can share with their doctor to enable more informed conversations.

And this isn't just about the individual. The benefits will also be seen at larger levels be they corporations, communities or societies. For businesses who encourage healthier practices, it could save thousands in sick days. For health services, the savings are potentially staggering. For each average stay in hospital, the financial costs are approximately $10,000 according to the agency for Healthcare Research and Quality. If mobile-enabled monitoring or diagnosis can reduce trips to the ER or reduce readmissions, then the savings will very quickly run into billions of dollars and companies old and new will rush to capture a slice of this very lucrative market.

New Players

If you were to ask most people to name the world's most powerful medical company, they would probably struggle. A few might mention big pharma brands like Pfizer, GSK or retailers such as CVS and Walgreens, but I would bet not many would say Apple or Google. Yet these two ostensibly technology giants are already targeting to be among the biggest players in health in the future. They are the gatekeepers to the smartphone world and recognize the potential for smartphones and associated technologies to change our lives dramatically. Without question, new leaders will emerge in the race for dominance of this consumer space, as the once insurmountable barriers to the health industry come tumbling down. I also expect to see consolidation with frequent mergers and acquisitions as distinct apps combine to create multi-purpose apps, competitors buy each other out and new players enter the fray.

Getting a Head Start

There's a lot to take in here. But rather than viewing the range of possibilities as intimidating, it's best to see it as a chance to find the solution that fits your personal needs and will help you maximize your well-being without a disproportionate effort. Few other technologies in history promise such a personally important dividend as the opportunity to improve your well-being. By adopting just some of the behaviors outlined in this book, you can get a head start on genuinely making positive strides towards a better lifestyle.

The pressure for choosing a proactive approach to health will grow dramatically - insurance company incentives, personal awareness of what's possible, health services struggling to cope, cost pressures, increased abilities of technologies, medical professionals and advisors embracing technology and recommending it to their patients - all these factors will push the adoption of the available technologies, and spur the development of even more innovations.

The speed at which technology is emerging is daunting, even for people who work in the industry full time. It is crossing traditional boundaries, challenging traditional ways of doing business and traditional roles. The focus of this book has not been on the technology per se. I do not believe that most people need to become experts in either their health or in the technologies available. But I do believe they have much to gain by developing sufficient awareness of changes that may be of benefit to them.

For some people it may be hard to take smartphones seriously as credible life saving devices. Following an early focus on camera prowess and social status updates, smartphones that have "matured" to offers apps such as Angry Birds and self-destructing Snapchats may not seem like potential life savers. But the sheer versatility enabled by the power of the smartphone to process, connect and display information makes it the ideal companion. The range of phone models combined with the sheer volume of apps, coupled with the further expansive possibilities of accessories could overwhelm even the most dedicated individual trying to decide where to start. Making a positive change to your lifestyle with your phone can begin in less time than it takes to top-up a prepaid device. As a starting point, I recommend you review the list of all the apps mentioned throughout this book, consolidated in Appendix A, and see which you might benefit from.

Sensible Choices - Consider How YOU Can Benefit

As we've seen, there is pretty much a sensor for every part of your body, and in many cases, several sensors that perform similar functions. Indeed, if you were to wear one of each available types of sensors, you would end up being covered in them, requiring near permanent electricity supply and devoting a huge amount of time to ensuring your phone synchronized with each one and trying to determine if any particular part of your anatomy needed attention, not to mention looking pretty ridiculous! Some of the more specific/niche technologies may sound a little gimmicky or improbable to you. If so, all I ask is that you remember that not all technologies are relevant for everyone and it's better to make a conscious decision that something isn't relevant to you than miss out through a lack of awareness.

As with so many things, the best approach to technology and health-related apps is to exercise moderation. Remember that some levels of detail provided by these technologies will only be of interest to serious athletes or people with chronic conditions. I am not advocating turning ordinary people into full time patients but we are at a turning point where it's now possible to have your phone act as a well-being advisor and guide, without requiring you to spend any money - so surely it's worth trying? If you are open to improving your well-being, do your research on the available options (where hopefully this book will help) and then consult your medical professional to discuss if any of the available options is recommended or particularly suited to your individual needs and circumstances.

It can be hard to see what's happening when you're in the midst of a revolution and it's tempting to wait to decide what to do until it all becomes clear. But the risk of that approach is that you are paralyzed into inactivity. So rather than sit idly by and miss out on any benefits available now until the more certain benefits have been determined, it seems a better approach to equip yourself with enough knowledge to make an informed decision on how much or how little you want to participate.

What, Where and When to Buy

I do hope I've demystified the multitude of solutions available and maybe even helped you develop an interest in one or more of the areas under discussion. There is no one-size fits all approach, either in terms of the apps and accessories available, or the motivations that people will have in turning to technology to assist them. So whether you're looking to prevent illness through better lifestyle or manage a chronic condition more effectively, you are best placed to know where your interest lies. You're more likely to succeed if you start small. Then, if you make one positive change, see if there's another you can layer on top of that.

As health and well-being technologies proliferate, and consumer interest in them develops, you'll see lots more examples hitting the high streets, online shops and app stores of the world. It can lead to some strange juxtapositions as blood-pressure monitors find their new home on shelves of supermarkets that are also selling food guaranteed to raise your blood pressure! But consumers will face purchasing decisions that bring medical-grade knowledge far closer to them than ever before as technology moves out of specialist shelves and onto mainstream shelves - e.g. blood pressure monitors are now available in a consumer electronics outlet at the airport, not just in a pharmacy.

I am often asked by friends who aren't especially interested in technology if there's a good time to buy a piece of technology that has piqued their curiosity. Perhaps they've been burnt before buying a model that is out of date just a few weeks after their proud acquisition but the reality is there is always likely to be a new improved model around the corner and there is probably no perfect time to buy if you want to have the latest gadget just for the sake of having the latest. My advice is to buy when you see a device or app that seems to meet your needs. Yes, it may be somewhat obsolete in a few months but the point of this is not to have the latest gadget - the point is to have a gadget that works for you, that makes a meaningful improvement in your life more possible, or less impossible, than it would be without the technical assistance.

And, happily, an increasingly common trend now is for devices to receive significant feature updates via software during their lifetime and you can in some cases expect them to improve hugely during their lifetime - and that's a lifetime measured in months or maybe a year or two! For example, the Alivecor device for ECG measurements mentioned in Chapter 3 has had two significant updates in less than a year - first gaining the ability to detect atrial fibrillation and secondly the ability to show Beat Fluctuation, a measure of how much the heartbeat changes from beat to beat.

It is undoubtedly hard to find the time in your day for all this. It will require discipline and inevitably comes with choices, priority calls and sacrifices. A growing number of people do persevere, aided by their will power and supported by technology. Make no mistake about it, there would not be the countless thousands of apps produced around fitness if there was not a market out there for them.

While there are immediate, practical and affordable steps you can take today to improve your health outlook with or without your phone, your well-being is not an isolated entity. It takes place in context - where technologies, data, human factors and policies will all intertwine. And while I would urge you to focus on the elements within your control, I feel it's important to highlight the wider context and bigger issues that are at play as this revolution unfolds.

Anyone embarking on lifestyle changes, based on the kinds of tracking technologies outlined earlier, should not be surprised if a doctor is not interested in your every movement. There may be a difference between what's interesting to you and what's useful to your doctor. They will likely only be interested in data that relates to your health and the problem you're presenting with. It may be interesting to you that you sleep less the days you have a lot of caffeine, but it's not medically significant in most cases. So remember that not all data is equal - your doctor is far more likely to be interested in high blood pressure readings for example, than your cadence.

Remember too, if you are an early adopter of these technologies, that the medical profession's response is still evolving, as is the technology itself, the regulatory framework and the healthcare administration frameworks necessary to exploit these changes. Overly enthusiastic technology advocates sometimes forget the very real challenges medical professionals face - life and death decisions, the inherent uncertainty and probabilities of medicine, along with the intangible social and human aspects. For their part, medical professionals should look to collaborate with technologists to unlock the potential on offer rather than quickly dismiss what may be the next breakthrough the equivalent of hygiene or the stethoscope for their profession.

Impacts on the Medical Profession

Despite the momentous changes, medicine as a discipline is not being threatened. In fact, it is being elevated and extended, supported by data scientists, technologists and even patients all collaborating to develop new ways to solve problems. At the heart of this trend is mobile technology - either in the form of sensors, or phones connected to massively powerful cloud and supercomputer systems that can help medical professionals with unprecedented resources always at their fingertips. Health care will now be continuous, anytime, anywhere and on-demand; not episodic and only in the local doctor's office. Many doctors are perhaps wary of the amateurization of their profession, unsure about technologies they don't fully understand and have little control over, as well as a public who frequently believe in both in miracle cures and the accuracy of anything they read on the Internet. That's why it's important to have an informed and inclusive debate on how, when and where technology should be adopted.

Change is not always easy in medicine. When Doctor Ignaz Semmelweis in Vienna in the mid 19th century proposed that doctors should wash their hands between carrying out autopsies and patient examinations, and that they should discard blood-stained clothes rather than wear them as a badge of authority, it was seen as an affront to doctors. Instead, his advice was what we later came to recognize as the emergence of hygienic medical practice.

In reading books such as "Do No Harm" and "Complications" which document what it's like to be a surgeon, you can't help but gain tremendous respect for medical professionals and the challenges they face with the potentially disastrous consequences of their fallibility. Yet the phrase "Doctors are human like the rest of us" may soon not be completely true. While humans remain better than machines at many tasks, robotic surgeons are increasingly performing operations. Human doctors can now be supported by the vast knowledge processing capabilities of machines and no longer have to rely solely on their experience or the extent of their reading ability to keep up with every medical development, test or theory in the world. I for one would rather they are assisted by the best medical computers in the world, accessible through the doctor's smartphone.

But it's important that we remain aware of the human aspects of medicine and never forget this reference from the modern version of the hippocratic oath: "I will remember that there is art to medicine as well as science, and that warmth, sympathy, and understanding may outweigh the surgeon's knife or the chemist's drug."

If mobile devices enable people to monitor their vital signs, conduct tests, provisionally diagnose diseases at home and communicate remotely with their doctors, then much of the current health infrastructure in developed countries becomes potentially unnecessary. At the very least, such a shift would remove pressure from overloaded hospitals and clinics. Meanwhile, the need for routine doctor visits plunges. Hospitals might be needed only for the acutely ill and for emergencies or operations or even, as Scripps's Dr Topol suggests, in their present form be "on their way out over time". Better monitoring and care might also eliminate the need for many drug prescriptions, cutting into the bottom line for pharmaceutical companies. One thing is clear - the scale and scope of the changes underway will have significant implications for the entire industry and Federal policies.

Impacts on Policies and Payers

The legislation that created the UK's National Health Service (NHS) set out a vision of: "a comprehensive health service designed to secure improvement in the physical and mental health of the people... and the prevention, diagnosis and treatment of illness". Over time, the majority of spending has come to be in the order: treatment, diagnosis and prevention, even though the original order might make more sense.

In most industrialized countries today, we have what is more correctly termed a sick-care system rather than healthcare. The majority of resources are directed towards caring for those that are already ill, rather than on preventing illness. Governments under increasing pressure to curb rising health costs will have to take tough decisions on prioritizing spending. But there aren't as many votes in preventative measures - it is often politically more expedient to provide a service that treats people when they are ill rather than be seen to be imposing draconian policies or restrictions on enjoyable or popular lifestyle choices.

The ageing populations of most nations will place unprecedented burdens on their health systems as people live longer but under the shadow of more chronic ailments. And to be blunt, ailments that in many cases will be the direct result of conscious bad health choices when information and assistance to avoid them were readily available. We are probably headed for a future healthcare scenario in most countries where it's simply not sustainable to offer free healthcare for cases where there is contributory negligence. So cyclists without helmets, drivers without seatbelts, smokers, intoxicated people and those who don't take reasonable care of their well-being may find that the more responsible elements of society are less agreeable to fund their indulgences.

Health insurers may take the lead and incentivize people to reduce avoidable illness - customers who do not show at least a reasonable level of care for their own health will likely be forced to pay extra. Any recourse to claims of ignorance, from people who choose not to better manage their well-being, will not be acceptable as medical information availability and quality increase, affordability of supportive technology improves and access to professional opinions becomes available on demand, 24x7.

Or if that sounds dystopian, then let me frame it another way - health insurance may become prohibitively expensive for people who choose not to take reasonable precautions. Of course accidents will still happen. People will fall ill despite their very best efforts. I am in no way suggesting that services for these people be curtailed. But I am expecting a debate in the coming years about the merits of providing care to people who choose behaviors they know are detrimental to their health yet expect others to pick up the tag when the foreseeable outcome happens sooner or later.

Policy makers in this new paradigm need to balance the theoretical improvements enabled by technology with the social and operational challenges in the real world. We also need to fix the existing anomalies that border on the absurd - healthcare insurance plans that are not interested in prevention because benefits may accrue to a future health insurer (given people switch providers on average every three years) as well as doctors and hospitals incentivized to see patients or operate on patients for additional payments rather than efficient outcomes. Despite the herculean efforts of many workers in the healthcare system and the emergence of technology that borders on the science fiction/magical, the barriers of policy must be addressed. It is disheartening in the extreme to read stories like this in the Economist:

> *Princess Alexandra Hospital, in Harlow, offers a new test for whether cancer has spread. The test, performed immediately after a lymph-node is removed, gives results in 40 minutes, rather than two weeks, which then allows other affected lymph-nodes to be taken out within the same operation. Malignant cancer needs a fast response. Yet only a handful of hospitals have adopted the test. According to the IPPR, this is partly because hospitals are paid per operation, and the test would mean one fewer.*

America's Affordable Care Act, better known as Obamacare, finally introduces penalties for hospitals when patients have to be readmitted and limits the sums hospitals can charge for certain conditions.

The economics of modern medicine are also worth keeping in mind. I don't want to sound paranoid, or to negate the huge benefits we have derived from pharmaceuticals or private hospitals, but there are some companies that do not especially want to see you well. They can extract additional profits by extending or exaggerating your condition or even creating new conditions. They create new variants of existing medicines not solely to increase efficacy or patient benefit but to increase patent duration. Business models in healthcare will be closely examined and likely be forced to change as disruptive technologies empower and democratize. But powerful interests and lobby groups will obfuscate and delay, often hiding behind emotive claims regarding patient safety.

Although not directly related to mobile technologies, these kinds of structural barriers to progress will become increasingly apparent as technology changes the rest of the healthcare sector and they will look all the more absurd. It is easier said than done, but vested interests of commercial hospitals, drug companies and health insurers will have to adapt if the healthier outcomes we desire are to come to fruition. The alliance of different interests has historically given rise to great progress. The Internet we take for granted today would likely not exist were it not for the cooperation of a military industrial academic complex of the 1960s. Similarly, it will take an unlikely cooperation of commercial, medical and government interests (with the willing participation of civilians) to deliver a higher quality of life for all.

Your Health and Politics

Health is a topic that should matter to all of us. But it's hard to prioritize it if you're in good health. It should be at or near the top of the list of things you care about when politicians come to canvass your vote. Better yet, your concern that medical services be improved should compel you to seek out your politicians and challenge them, rather than wait until you need health care only to discover it's below the standard you expect.

A recent report on the future of the health service in Ireland noted:

"Health is more than merely the absence of disease; it is physical, mental, and social well-being. Most common chronic diseases, disabilities and injuries can be prevented. Investments in prevention complement and support treatment and care. Prevention policies and programmes can be cost-effective, can reduce healthcare costs, and can improve the health of the population.

Health is also a key factor in productivity, economic development and growth. The role of the health service must be seen as keeping people healthy as opposed to just treating sick people. Overall, health reform must lead to a healthy Ireland where health and wellbeing is valued by all individuals at every level of society, is embraced by every sector and is everyone's responsibility."

It's hard to disagree with any of that but I find the final two words among the most interesting - a vision that firmly expands responsibility to include the individual. But if you expect it to be everyone's responsibility, you have to provide them with the information and tools to understand their choices and options and inputs. It also begs the question about where the line between responsibility and compulsion/enforcement will be drawn. This is where some of the biggest decisions need to be made regarding mobile and associated technologies.

Mandating Technology?

"If people let the government decide what foods they eat and what medicines they take, their bodies will soon be in as sorry a state as are the souls who live under tyranny."

- Thomas Jefferson

Larry Smarr, a professor of computer science at the University of California at San Diego, has spent 15 years studying his vital signs and activities before the current generation of devices for this purpose was even imaged, let alone available. He believes that these devices and tests will help people take personal responsibility for their own health. His experience reinforces the notion that these devices remove any barriers to people taking more responsibility for their own well-being. "The mythology in this country is you can do whatever you want to your body, and a doctor will give you a pill to fix it. That needs to change," Smarr said.

In most progressive societies, we generally agree that people should be free to do as they choose in their personal lives. Where it becomes more complicated is if the consequences of those choices impact on others. In the case of health choices, that impact is already being seen in the spiraling costs of healthcare. In essence, people making poor choices are expecting others to pay for their choices. And as technology exposes the extent of preventable illness, and provides ever-better means of assisting prevention, I believe tough decisions lie ahead about the acceptability of choosing not to adopt healthier lifestyle choices.

I am not advocating to take the fun out of life - there are no guarantees no matter how 'healthy' your lifestyle regime is. The kinds of lifestyle choices we should be making are fairly widely known, even if they are not widely embraced. In most cases, we've known for many years what healthier lifestyles and diets are and, as the growth of chronic illnesses shows, we've largely ignored them. Even as our understanding grows of why a high fiber diet is actually good for controlling weight (it's to do with bacteria called Bacteroidetes and Firmicutes among others if you're interested), it doesn't change the long-standing recommendation to eat more fiber.

What's changed is that ignoring existing knowledge used be more easily justified as monitoring and managing one's own health was prohibitively difficult. But technology has removed so many barriers - apps for awareness and education, accessories to track our exercise and even what we eat - all are available, affordable, accessible and improving continuously. Yet a substantial proportion of the population will have to adapt these practices to stem the healthcare cost crisis. If the pull of the promise of significantly reduced risk of chronic illness and even death is not sufficient, attention will inevitably turn to the push factors - financial and other inducements.

As tools to manage your own well-being become more widely available, we may see those who do embrace personal responsibility begin to resent paying taxes to fund a health service for people who don't? Lynne Dunbrack, who covers personal monitoring devices and related areas as research vice president for IDC Health Insights points out that with a few exceptions, "consumers just aren't that interested in managing their health or reviewing their health records that closely". Sacrifice is not popular, and without a clear near-term incentive, people are unlikely to take action that may benefit them in the long term. As author Gabe Zichermann puts it: "Fundamentally, people are bad at deferring pleasure now for future gain and avoidance of pain. I liken it to pensions. It's something we know we should have when we're young but the lack of an immediate return makes it hard to prioritize. And unlike pensions, there's not the hope of a windfall inheritance that will change things. Ultimately as health insurers and care-givers impose additional fees for those who do not take shared responsibility, it will be your personal perspective as to whether this is an incentive or a penalty."

Trolleyology

Borrowing from psychology, I wonder if we may need to apply the concepts of Trolleyology to decisions in healthcare. Posed by moral philosopher Philippa Foot in 1967, this thought experiment has many variants but essentially deals with this conundrum: Standing on a footbridge overlooking a railway track, an observer sees a trolley hurtling toward five people tied to the rails. Next to her is a very fat man, who, if pushed onto the track, would stop the trolley before it reached the quintet. Would you – should you – kill one fat man to save five lives?

Adapting this puzzle to modern healthcare and the potential changes enabled by mobile technologies, should we consider forcing people to lead healthier lives so as to free up resources for the greater good? While not faced with pushing the proverbial fat man onto the track, should we force the fat man to take steps to become slim? Is it morally acceptable to continue to spend on avoidable problems to the detriment of research? Are we guilty of failing to act to save people? I don't propose to answer the question here but I foresee debate about the resourcing and priority decisions that are coming down the tracks towards us, much like the trolley in the experiment.

The Dividend

Although the human benefits are immense, in the shape of avoided or postponed ill health potentially enabled by adopting mobile technologies, it is likely that the direct and indirect financial benefits that could accrue will be the driving force behind the broader adoption of mobile well-being technologies. Extending beyond the current worried well cohort into the population at large is where it can help to address spiraling healthcare costs.

A recent PwC report estimated that mobile health technology adoption could save 99 billion EUR in healthcare costs in the European Union (EU) and add 93 billion EUR to the EU GDP in 2017. Those sort of headline grabbing numbers will pique interest among hard-pressed health departments, but to look at it in human terms instead of money, the same report highlights the opportunity to help 185 million patients lead healthier lives and gain 158,000 years of life. We tend to think of our health in very personal terms, but the cumulative impact on a society of diseases and lifestyle choices is huge - by 2017, around 70 million chronic patients could lose up to 718 billion EUR in wages due to around 60 billion work hours lost in absenteeism and early retirement.

The McKinsey Global Institute concentrated a chapter of its report "The Internet of Things: Mapping the Value Beyond the Hype 2015" on health matters, concluding with an overall estimate that the use of these technologies in human health applications could have an economic impact of $171 billion to $1.6 trillion globally in 2025. The report highlighted the economic and operational benefits of connected technologies for more continuous and consistent monitoring of patients with chronic diseases to help patients avoid medical crises, hospitalizations, and complications.

Similarly, Accenture noted in another recent report that digital health offerings can drive more than $100 billion in savings over that same time period to 2018 and saved the US healthcare system $6 billion last year in the form of improved medication adherence, behavior modifications and fewer emergency room visits.

Embracing the Technology

Leaving behind the larger scale political and policy stage to return to the discussion of how to best understand the emerging technologies, there are two theoretical models that are especially useful in understanding the uptake of new developments and innovations. New technologies coming to the market follow stages of what Gartner call the "Hype Cycle" - from their initial invention, through enthusiastic proclamations that they are a panacea, to a realization they may not be everything that was initially promised to a gradual emergence and settling at their eventual uptake and impact level. Depending on your perspective as a consumer, healthcare professional, researcher or policymaker, your view of where these technologies currently sit on the axis may be different. That's ok and I'm not expecting everyone to agree on an exact location along the curve for every product - what I am adamant we need though, is awareness, discussion and informed choices on each of those levels - from individuals and medical professionals through to researchers and policy makers. Only then will we see a realistic progression along the axis towards the maximum benefits that are possible.

From a consumer point of view, the "Diffusion of Innovations" theory splits consumers into five broad groups - from innovators through to laggards who have different interest levels in adopting technologies and will do so at a different pace. The various technologies in this book will see different rates of progress along these two models. Some of the areas discussed will perhaps never emerge from the trough of disillusionment or see adoption outside of innovators. Yet we will see some technologies adopted by people we would otherwise consider laggards due to a personal or family interest in a specific relief.

Silver Bullet?

So is technology the solution to the challenges of making society healthy while balancing the books? It holds great potential to help advance healthcare and societal well-being, it is not the sole answer to all ills. Pun intended.

Despite the promise of improvements, poor implementations of technology are often no better than no technology at all. The book, "The Digital Doctor", chronicles the disappointments and missteps of the roll-out of Electronic Health Records (EHR) backed by a $30bn dollar government fund in the US to show that improperly applied, technology is not the answer. Technology is a promising enabler that will succeed only if used sensibly and deployed with a healthy mix of technical, medical, commercial and political involvement.

And Finally...

Our most important challenge is to envision the future we want and set about bringing it to fruition - not to passively predict its predetermined path and complain if we aren't happy with the outcome.

The innovation in technology for our well-being will continue, the accuracy will improve, the prices will decrease and the functionality will merge into ever more convenient form factors. Relentless technological advances have brought cost reduction and miniaturization that have made it possible to completely rethink which technologies can be consumerized will bring more unimaginable diagnostic powers to our pockets.

In the book "The Second Machine Age", the authors declared "It is no exaggeration to say that billions of people will soon have a printing press, reference library, school and computer all at their fingertips". However, what the authors didn't mention is consultant, trainer, clinic or laboratory, which we also now can have. They did highlight the importance of combinatorial progress and I believe their findings apply especially to healthcare's future - rather than a single vertical industry breakthrough, healthcare's future will involve collaborative and combinatorial advances.

Little more than a generation ago, infectious diseases such as measles, smallpox and polio killed millions of people every year. Thankfully now those ailments are a distant memory in most of the world, new threats such as diabetes, heart disease and obesity are this generation's killers. Just as previous seminal medical breakthroughs such as antibiotics, hospital hygiene and vaccinations saved countless lives, the application of technology to tackle today's medical challenges will be a watershed moment. Inevitably, the medical profession will adapt and adopt, while patients will choose to embrace or ignore. In any event, the consumerization of medicine and the medicalization of consumers will rapidly gain pace.

The shift towards mobile is accelerating. And there are other adjacent changes that will modify the medical landscape - there are now Internet-based mail order services for Biome and DNA testing that add to the data but place further pressures on the medical profession and regulators to manage expectations. Although the pace of change is already astounding, we are still in the early stages of parallel, simultaneous revolutions. The same and related smart technologies that are impacting healthcare are gaining momentum in creating smart homes and smart cities that will turn our very near future into lifestyles that closely resemble science-fiction predictions.

2015 feels like a seminal year in this revolution. Yes many of the devices and applications are not yet ready for prime time and very much resemble version one products. And yes, many doctors, people and patients are not yet aware of or ready to embrace the changes that lie ahead. It's not all plain sailing - The possibilities of these new and emerging technologies are countered by risks, including the potential for privacy issues, misdiagnosis and more.

The pace of change will likely quicken before levelling off. But the incentive to invest some time in researching and harnessing the technology available to improve your well-being should prove great enough for most people to at least consider it. What I hope is that there are some apps or accessories mentioned here that you suspect may help you to make a change towards a somewhat healthier lifestyle, without sacrificing too much of what you enjoy.

The last century has seen the greatest single improvement in life expectancy in most countries in the history of civilization - medical advances, infrastructure advances and nutrition have combined to enable leaps in longevity. Reductions in infant mortality, improvements in health and safety along with health insurance have had a dramatic positive impact. The imminent mobile technology revolution can continue to deliver gains and reverse the setbacks of the latter half of the 20th century; make no mistake that every year of life increase matters on a personal level, even if it is not as statistically significant. It's vital we remember that these are people we are talking about, not just numbers. If we don't take full advantage of the new tools at our disposal, we face being the first generation since records began to live less than the previous one.

I genuinely believe we are lucky to be alive at a time of this perfect storm of hardware, software, entrepreneurship - giving us affordable hardware, miniaturization, available computing power, and connectivity. This new world comes with opportunity and peril in differing measures, partly dependent on one's perspective, awareness and partly on how the technologies are implemented. A lack of understanding at policy and government level threatens to leave gaps, while the medical professional faces a challenge of unprecedented scale and will play a pivotal role in both guiding and maximizing this era.

Your personal trainer, medic, nutritionist, psychologist, therapist and cardiologist can all now be a simple tap or swipe away. That's not to exclude your mindfulness mentor, dentist and environmental expert. Given the power at our fingertips to extend and improve our lives, we only have ourselves to blame if we let the opportunity to harness it slip away. Your phone really can save your life.

Appendices

Appendix A: Technologies Mentioned

This appendix contains a list of the products, apps and services mentioned in this book. This is not an endorsement or recommendation, but provided as a convenience if you'd like further information on any specific product. The full list and accompanying links is provided on the book's web site at http://www.yourphonecansaveyourlife.com

Products

Product	Style	Features
Up 3	Wristband	Activity/Sleep/HR
Up 4	Wristband	Activity/Sleep/HR
Up Move	Clip-on/Wristband	Activity/Sleep
Healbe	Wrist Band	Calories, Activity, Sleep, HR and Blood Pressure
Apple Watch	Smartwatch	Activity/HR
Android Wear	Smartwatch	Activity/HR
Misfit Shine	Clip-on/Wristband	Activity, Sleep
Moov	Wristband	Activity
LG Lifeband	Wristband	Activity
LG Headphones	Headphones	HR
Sony Smartband Talk	Smartwatch	Activity/Sleep
Basis Peak	Smartwatch	Activity/Sleep/HR

Polar Flow	Wristband	Activity/Sleep
Garmin Vivo	Wristband	Activity/Sleep
Fitbit Flex	Wristband	Activity/Sleep
Garmin HR Monitor	Chest Strap	HR
Polar HR Monitor	Chest Strap	HR
Ampstrip	Adhesive	HR
Withings Pulse	Clip on/Wristband	Activity/Sleep/HR/Pulse Ox
Alivecor	Accessory	ECG, HR
Jabra HR Headphones	Headphones	HR
Microsoft Band	Smartwatch	Activity, Sleep, HR
Scanadu Scout	Accessory	Temperature, HR, Blood Pressure, Pulse Ox
Withings Body Analyzer	Scales	Weight, BMI, Fat %
iHealth Core Scale	Scales	Weight, BMI, Fat %s
Clinicloud	Accessory	Temperature and Lung Sounds
Spire	Clip-on	Activity & Stress
Kito Azoi	Accessory	HR
Scanadu Urine	Accessory	Urine Checks
Cue	Accessory	Mini Lab
MinION	Accessory	Portable DNA
Samsung Gear Fit	Smartwatch	Activity, Sleep, HR
Sensoria Socks	Clothing/Accessory	Activity

MiBand	Wristband	Activity, Sleep
Fitbit Tony Burch	Wristband	As per Fitbit Flex
Misfit Swarovski	Wristband	As per Misfit Shine
Hexoskin	Clothing/Accessory	
Prepad	Accessory	Food Weight
HidrateMe	Accessory	Liquid Consumption
Vessyl	Accessory	Liquid Composition
Hapi Fork	Accessory	Eating Pace
BitBite	Ear piece	Eating Pace
Food Sniffer	Accessory	Food Quality
TellSpec	Accessory	Food Composition
Beddit	Accessory	Sleep, HR
Withings Aura	Accessory	Sleep, HR, Luminosity, Sounds, Room Temperature
Sense	Accessory	Sleep
S+	Accessory	Sleep, Luminosity, Room Temperature
PIP	Accessory	Stress
MUSE	Headband	Stress
Blucub	Accessory	Room Temperature, Humidity
Nest Thermostat	Accessory	Room Temperature
Nest Protect	Accessory	Smoke, CO_2 and CO
Netatmo Weather Station	Accessory	Room Temperature, Air Quality, humidity

Withings Home	Accessory	VOC
Air Mentor Pro	Accessory	Air Quality
Netatmo June	Wristband	UV
Violet	Clip-on	UV
Sunsprite	Clip-on	UV
Wave	Accessory	Skin
OKU	Accessory	Skin
Lumo Lift	Clip-on	Posture, Activity
Darma	Accessory	Posture
Oral B	Accessory	Brushing
Kolibree	Accessory	Brushing
Breathometer Mint	Accessory	Oral Health, Breath Quality
Cellscope	Accessory	Ear health
Vitastiq	Accessory	Vitamin & Mineral Levels
AMPY	Accessory	Charging

Apps

Name	Category
Vital Signs	HR, Breathing Rate
ResApp	Respiration
Theranos	Blood Testing Locations/Results
CityMapper	Calories used by different transport choices
Spotify	Music
Audible	Audiobooks
LifeSum	Food Intake
MFP	Food Intake
Foodswitch	Food Substitution recommendations
Fooducate	Food Education
HapiCoach	Personal Coach
Rise	Personal Coach
Lark	Personal Coach
Sleep Better with Runtastic	Sleep
Jawbone Up Coffee	Caffeine Tracking
Twilight	Sleep
Headspace	Meditation
Calm	Meditation
Lumosity	Brain Training
Peak	Brain Training

Exist	Mood Management
Pacifica	Mood Management
5Min Journal	Mind Clearance
Backup Memory	Dementia Support
Sunwise	UV
DMinder	Sun
SunZapp	Sun
Eyecare Plus	Eye Tests
ViaOpta Daily	Visual Impaired Help
ViaOpta Nav	Visual Impaired Help
ViaOpta Simulator	Visual Impaired Simulation
Noise Meter App	Sound Levels
Hearing App	Auditory Performance
MyMeds	Adherence
Medisafe	Adherence
Walgreens	Pharmacy & Medicine Services
CVS	Pharmacy & Medicine Services
Atari Fit	Activity/Gamification
Matchup	Activity Challenges
Pact	Paid Activity Challenges
Zombies, Run!	Activity/Gamification
The Walk	Activity/Gamification
WebMD	Medical Information
Patients Like Me	Patient Community

Iodine	Drug Information
Folding@home	Donate Processing Power
Powertogive	Donate Processing Power
GoodSAM	Volunteer First Responder
MyDirectives	End of Life Medical Preferences
Medscape	Professional Medical Information
Epocrates	Professional Medical Information
UpToDate	Professional Medical Information
Isabel	Professional Medical Information
Doximity	Medical Network
Figure1	Professional Medical Information
Apscript	Professional Medical Information
Zocdoc	Doctor Look-up service
Babylon	Virtual Doctor
Your.MD	Virtual Doctor
Dr On Demand	Virtual Doctor
iTriage	Medical Information
ZipDrug	Prescription Delivery Service
Quealth	Health Assessment
MedXNote	Professional Medical Messaging
Gauss Surgical	Professional Medical Blood Absorption
Addapp	Health Insights
Dacadoo	Health Aggregation
Fluview	Mapping Influenza Like Illness

SickWeather	Mapping Illnesses
Healthyday	Mapping Illnesses
Nutrimatix	Supplement advice
Wellpath	Supplement advice
UnderArmour	Exercise

Web Services

Name	Category
Lumoid	Tracker Trials
Flaredown	Chronic Illness Monitoring
Smartpatients.com	Health Community
zenobase.com	Health Aggregation
Tictrac	Health Insights
Omadahealth.com	Corporate Well-being
23andme	Genetic testing
uBiome	Microbiotics

Appendix B: Reading & References

I've included references here to some of the key texts I used during my research for this book. A more complete list is available on the web site at: http://www.yourphonecansaveyourlife.com

Books

- Do No Harm: Stories of Life, Death and Brain Surgery - Henry Marsh

- Bad Science - Ben Goldacre

- Testing Treatments: Better Research for Better Healthcare - Imogen Evans, Hazel Thornton, Iain Chalmers, Paul Glasziou, Ben Goldacre

- The Drugs Don't Work (Penguin Special): A Global Threat (Penguin Shorts/Specials) - Professor Dame Sally Davies, Jonathan Grant, Mike Catchpole

- Complications: A Surgeon's Notes on an Imperfect Science - Atul Gawande

- Bad Pharma: How Medicine is Broken, And How We Can Fix It - Ben Goldacre

- Digital Disruption: Unleashing the Next Wave of Innovation - James McQuivey, Josh Bernoff

- Age of Context: Mobile, Sensors, Data and the Future of Privacy - Robert Scoble, Shel Israel

- The Patient Will See You Now: The Future of Medicine is in Your Hands - Eric Topol

- Connected Health: How Mobile Phones, Cloud and Big Data Will Reinvent Healthcare - Jody Ranck

- The Creative Destruction of Medicine: How the Digital Revolution Will Create Better Health Care - Eric Topol

- Smart Cities: Big Data, Civic Hackers, and the Quest for a New Utopia - Anthony M. Townsend

- The Digital Doctor: Hope, Hype, and Harm at the Dawn of Medicine's Computer Age - Robert Wachter

- Would You Kill the Fat Man? - David Edmonds

- The Making of Modern Medicine - BBC Audiobooks

- Overdiagnosed: Making People Sick in Pursuit of Health - H. Gilbert Welch, Lisa M. Schwartz,Steven Woloshin

- 10% Human - How Your Body's Microbes Hold the Key to Health and Happiness - Alanna Collen

- 'Better Doctors, Better Patients, Better Decisions: Envisioning Health Care 2020 (Strüngmann Forum Reports)

- Where Does It Hurt?: An Entrepreneur's Guide to Fixing Health Care - Jonathan Bush, Stephen Baker

- Automate This: How Algorithms Came to Rule Our World - Christopher Steiner

- The Marshmallow Test – Walter Mischel